KUNO
VAN DER POST

MISSING LINKS IN HEALING

*A NEW-OLD
APPROACH FOR A
CHAOTIC WORLD*

ISBN: 978-1-7637862-6-4 (paperback)

A catalogue record for this
book is available from the
National Library of Australia

Cover art by Anze Ban Virant
Printed and distributed by Ingram Spark
Published by Kuno van der Post
missinglinksbook@proton.me

Contents

Introduction

If I told you there is a cure for shingles—one that is very cheap, highly effective, with no serious danger and no lasting consequences—what would you think?

It must be a herb? A vitamin? A common drug with a benefit not widely known about? Or that it's too good to be true? The man's deluded? What can he possibly know that the best doctors and biomedical scientists don't? Or that I'm a con-merchant selling useless snake-oil for an unpleasant but otherwise not serious condition?

Who am I even to talk about these matters? I will come to that shortly.

The cure is this: wait a month. Yes, that's it. Nothing more, nothing less. The issue is not whether it will pass, it is the degree of suffering to be tolerated in the meantime. Waiting also works to a greater or lesser extent for countless other so-called 'conditions' such as colds, flu, indigestion, headaches, back pain, to name a few.

Of course, someone may be thinking, but hang on, you can't do that: somebody they knew had a serious complication or long-term harm from shingles, or even died. The question they should ask is whether medical treatment could have prevented those outcomes, and the answer is probably not [1] [2]. Death caused by shingles is rare—fewer than 100 cases a year in the USA [3]. You are at least 11 times more likely to be killed by an insect [4], 40 times more likely to drown [5], and 1000 times more likely to be killed by a prescribed drug [6]. I will argue

later why I think the drugs are, in fact, far more dangerous even than that.

So, let me see the case and ask enough questions, and I
will point you to where I think it was something else, perhaps less obvious than the illness, that probably caused
those more serious outcomes. There were likely many
other factors involved besides the illness itself.

Still, a discussion about healing needs more than that.
We need to talk about ways to alleviate suffering, and
there are ways. But we first need to lay the groundwork
for understanding the problems we are looking to solve,
how they come about, and what we are trying to achieve.
We need some kind of roadmap to guide us from A to B.

We need to consider why it is that we even need something better. What are the missing links that make modern healthcare, in all its forms, less than complete? Is it a
lack of funding for more breakthroughs? Or is it something more fundamental? And what do we even stand for
as practitioners?

These are some of the subjects I will explore in this
book. And in case it needed stating, the highest priority
remains that we don't make matters worse. The point of
healing is not just to relieve suffering, but to avoid lasting
harm overall. If that last is all we ever aim for as healers,
we might still turn out to be more effective than our com-
petitors would believe.

But we also really need to establish what we mean by
health and disease, and state some of our goals. In doing
so, we may discover that many of the problems we have
aren't really problems, that the solutions are right under
our own noses, or that we don't even need to have those

issues in the first place. As patients, we will still experience illness as bumps in the road, but we won't need to fear it halting our progress through life.

And who am I? I have science and healthcare degrees, but I'm not a scientific or medical expert. Some of my patients see me as an authority on health, but many of them are more up to date than me. I could do more exercise and eat more wisely. I struggle with bad habits and procrastination, the same as anybody, and I am prone to taking on far more stress than I would advise. I have enjoyed effortless good health for much of my life and suffered difficulties as well.

But through adversity, I discovered a knack for helping others get better, eventually qualifying as an osteopath and practicing in three countries. I am privileged to have accompanied many people on their successful journeys out of many kinds of trouble.

I began writing as a response to my own trauma, that of seeing my parents rendered helpless by the systems I once believed were there to give them back their independence. The real surprise, however, was seeing the helplessness of those systems. Medicine seemed imbued with a sense of unrequited hope, sprinkled with nuggets of comforting reassurance and the odd morsel of success. Having made some sense of that experience, the hope is I can use the lessons learned to help others see the sense in their own situation, whether they are suffering or in the position of guiding others through suffering. As a practitioner, one is both.

My father was a talented engineer, but he lived with terrible respiratory illness and a near constant bad back.

Those problems did not seem, at the time, to be related to each other, nor to the fact that he died from an aggressive cancer at fifty-five.

It took me another twenty years or so to recognise that it was probably medicine that killed him. It wasn't through any medical error or lack of care. His treatment was delivered with excellence. But it was brutal nevertheless, and the futility should have been obvious. It was that more modest treatment for a milder condition in his youth set the trajectory, and that terminal cancer was for him its destination. At no point was he offered another path.

There was at the time a sense of vital breakthroughs just around the corner. Even though the answers wouldn't come in time for my father, the silver lining was that others might be helped. Forty years later, it seems as if they are still just around the corner.

I never set out to be a healer. But life handed me three challenges, and with that, choices. Firstly, I broke my back in a parachuting accident. Luckily, I recovered easily, but it opened my mind to certain ideas.

Then, a few months later, my mother suffered from a brain haemorrhage, and was let down badly by a flagship medical rehabilitation centre. The terrible waste of potential we witnessed as a family set me on a path, and I began applying what I had learned through my injury, determined to do better for her. She proved the experts wrong and went on to enjoy a very productive life for nearly two decades; travelling overseas, hosting her own dinner parties, sitting on the village council, and being chased by men, before suffering a decline towards the end.

About two years after my mother's illness began, I feared I might lose my own health entirely. It was a brilliant alternative therapist in London who got me back on track. I realised there is no way my actual doctor would have even recognised the problem for what it was: I had been harmed by travel vaccines delivered at her own clinic.

After all that, there was no going back. My loss of faith through these events left a void, quickly filled by a realisation that there are other ways to do things—excellent ways—besides what we might call the medical way. And somehow, I ended up embarking on an exhausting five-year training in osteopathy. Even before I qualified, I began to have serious doubts about whether osteopathy itself was all it was supposed to be. My chosen field, once a serious medical discipline, seemed to have a lot of links missing, just as I had seen with modern medicine. Eventually, I would go looking for them.

Partly because of the excellent clinical education I received, and partly in defiance of it, I came to see the typical problems people came in with, as inseparable from the more general health baggage they often brought along as well. Finally, I came to realise, that health is the only workable solution to disease, and it doesn't work selectively.

Had I chosen to trust the experts, no doubt another equilibrium would have arrived, and I would have been just as happy. The one thing I did learn to trust was the ability of the human body to recover. If there is a moral to all this, it is that we have been told many half-truths about the way things work in our world, and that we must each find the truth within ourselves if we are to evolve as a species.

So, I don't have anything special to say about shingles in particular: it's just as good an entry point as any to a discussion about alternative medicine. What I hope to show is that one can deal with a great many health problems from a set of first principles, at times far more usefully than through the orthodox medical reasoning.

From time to time, people ask me what to do about shingles, and I always ask them why they think they need to do anything. Not only can a great many cases of illness do just fine without direct intervention, it can often be the better way to approach things. Hence, the skill of the great practitioner is knowing when to do something, when to leave things alone, and, from time to time, when the hospital really is needed.

And when practitioners act, do we seek to fix things as the hero of the day? Or do we see ours as a supporting role? The answer is, it depends, and the only way we can approach this in an unfamiliar situation is through those first principles. And I would argue that all cases are unfamiliar, in some way. Point one is, do no harm. Point two is trust the human body.

Navigating things from there takes a framework, and what I offer in these pages is both a personal critique of the reactive approach we have all learned to live with, and a fresh way of looking at things, for those who feel, as I do, that something has been missing from our healthcare. And I will start by explaining why this is desperately needed.

[1] Chen N, Li Q, Yang J, Zhou M, Zhou D, He L. *Antiviral treatment for preventing postherpetic neuralgia.* Cochrane Database of Systematic Reviews 2014, Issue 2. Art. No.: CD006866. DOI: 10.1002/14651858.CD006866.pub3.

[2] Jiang X, Li Y, Chen N, Zhou M, He L. *Corticosteroids for preventing postherpetic neuralgia.* Cochrane Database of Systematic Reviews 2023, Issue 12. Art. No.: CD005582. DOI: 10.1002/14651858. CD005582.pub5.

[3] *Shingles Facts and Stats,* CDC, https://www.cdc.gov/shingles/data-research/index.html.

[4] QuickStats: *Number of Deaths from Hornet, Wasp, and Bee Stings, Among Males and Females* — National Vital Statistics System, United States, 2000–2017. MMWR Morb Mortal Wkly Rep 2019; 68:649 .

[5] *Drowning facts,* CDC, https://www.cdc.gov/drowning/data-research/facts/index.html.

[6] Lazarou J, Pomeranz BH, Corey PN. *Incidence of adverse drug reactions in hospitalized patients: a meta-analysis of prospective studies.* JAMA. 1998 Apr 15;279(15):1200-5. doi: 10.1001/jama.279.15.1200. PMID: 9555760.

What are the missing links, where did they go, and how are we going to get them back?

Though the doctors treated him, let his blood, and gave him medications to drink, he nevertheless recovered.

—Leo Tolstoy

The range of pharmaceutical treatments available today is so absolutely mind-boggling ... who can keep up? It covers the familiar, day to day, over the counter (OTC) pills for things that nearly always get better on their own, right through to highly exotic chemicals for advanced disease costing thousands of dollars a pop. It is a moot point whether they actually cure anything. They can manage the symptoms, and in some cases can get us out of serious trouble. Some can help speed up the process of recovery or make the wait more bearable, but it is arguable they don't do much, if anything, to improve our actual health.

Since drugs are essentially tiny doses of poisons, they also risk making matters far worse, or prolonging the

problem, or setting one up for further episodes; risks
most people accept, since they are unaware of just how
common such negative outcomes are. Even good old
aspirin may be responsible for thousands of deaths per
year in the UK [1]. Should we be relying on medications
less than we are? I think so.

There are many remedies for a headache, and antacids and laxatives are major money spinners for pharmacies. All, or nearly all, of these everyday treatments are
for the symptoms only. And in many cases the symptoms
will go away on their own, assuming they don't signify
some more serious problem. The real challenge for the
great therapist or physician is not making these things go
away: it is stopping them from coming back, and without
the patient developing further problems and becoming
dependent on treatment.

Even antibiotics—supposedly the clearest example of
a drug cure—have been over relied upon, and in many
instances their benefits are questionable. Killing germs
directly can sometimes save lives, but the war on germs
has failed in the main objective of reducing the overall
burden of disease. I'll explain later that these drugs seem
to have altered the profile of the diseases we face, but not
made them go away. And that germs themselves, even
dangerous ones, are at most opportunists and not the
true cause of disease. The seeds of dangerous disease
have often been sown years before any germ shows up.

Most of the time when one has an infection, the body
still copes just fine, and resolves matters without help.
And when it occasionally doesn't, there are various ways
to turn things around without antibiotics, that can work

quite reliably. There are, of course, lives saved by antibiotics, and if all else fails, it is good to know they are there. But they can also make matters worse and cause severe and even fatal reactions as well.

Furthermore, they can't deal with the conditions that allow a so-called infection to take hold, and once they have stabilised the situation, the painstaking work of restoring health must begin. If that final step is not taken—and it usually isn't—then the patient is almost certainly on the road back towards some kind of health problem.

Many of the so-called risks of illness are, quite often, risks of the way they are managed. For solving a great many minor problems—and even some supposedly serious ones—much of the work of the therapist involves stopping the patient from doing anything silly. And for the patient and their advocates, it can mean stopping their doctors from doing anything unnecessary.

Even in emergency medicine, doing less may produce better results. Some intensive care experts believe less aggressive measures save more lives, even in those who are critically ill [2].

Numerous studies have shown that when doctors go on strike, death rates actually fall [3]. One remarkable survey in the United States even found that the longer it takes paramedics to reach you, the greater your chances of surviving a heart attack [4]. Such findings deserve considering from every possible angle, and we shouldn't take them at face value. But the assumption I would challenge is that heroic intervention is always helpful. I am certainly not advising against calling paramedics if you need them. But there is reason to think that a light touch and minimal intervention is occasionally more in line with what a sick person really needs.

True enough, there is great merit in addressing underlying causes. Later on, I will explain why causes are usually far more elusive than textbooks would tell us. I will argue that most therapies aimed at treating causes, more often than not, hit the nail squarely on the thumb.

But there are ways to support the body while it sorts things out. They generally work indirectly and without trying to actually fix things, since the body is already fixing itself through the expression of symptoms.

So, the big money in healing is in various forms of symptom management (palliation). And aggressive expert intervention to stabilise a situation can be of great value. But the clues to actual resolution are found elsewhere, in something very elusive, very hard to describe, virtually impossible to measure, namely health. And obtaining a thorough conceptual or practical handle on health seems to defeat some of the best brains in healthcare. To date, doctors can't even agree on a single definition for it. That, and the issues surrounding how we consider health and disease, is what this book is about.

Specifically, it is about concepts and thinking tools, as a lead in to how we structure actual treatment. It is intended to bridge a gap that was left in my own training: that is, the gap between natural healing ideals and actual clinical practice. It is certainly not meant as a practical guide, and there is no substitute for training or experience.

I don't suggest that serious health problems (or even mild ones) should go without being addressed, or that there is some puritanical reason for ignoring them. If I thought that, I'd be in the wrong business. But the fact is, *their causes* usually do go unaddressed, and we need to look at the subject of cause from a completely different point of view to the medical perspective, or even the mainstream of the so-called alternative offerings, in order to really deal with it.

Our health has been stolen from us and is being sold back as countless lucrative ways to manage the symptoms that result. This was partly an accident and partly a classic land grab. The American medical system was reformed just over a century ago, supposedly to bring it onto a sound, rational footing. But driving these reforms were the Rockefeller and the Carnegie Foundations, major stakeholders in the rapidly expanding chemical and drugs business. Their true purpose was to own the medical field and make a great deal of money. And they largely succeeded.

Those organisations went to great lengths to ensure doctors were trained to see all medical problems as a need for a drug, and to organise the hospitals as the means to deliver it. Medical schools and hospitals that didn't at least give primacy to this philosophy were effectively outlawed. Around the same time, the American Medical Association (AMA) became very active in marketing medical products, and more hostile towards therapies that might be seen as competition.

As *'A Midwestern Doctor'* puts it, the medical system that took shape in the early 1900s has worked tirelessly ever since to *"… promote healthy activities people are unlikely to do (e.g., exercising or smoking cessation) … promote clearly unhealthy activities industries make money from (e.g., eating processed foods or taking a myriad of unsafe and ineffective pharmaceuticals) …*

[and] attack clearly beneficial activities that are easy to do (e.g., sunlight exposure, eating eggs, consuming raw dairy, or eating butter)" [5].

Furthermore, it actively opposes rival theories and approaches [6].

The result is that hospitals—which are some of the most dangerous places that most of us will ever go—frequently offer little to benefit our health and just as likely set us up for the next visit. If they really were getting us healthy, they would be getting smaller, one might think. Instead, they get bigger and bigger, but disease is just as big a problem as ever—what you would expect from an effective repeat-business generation scheme.

Most of us have grown up to think rational medicine can only ever be this way. Even our language has been distorted to support this impression; the term 'side-effects' being just one example. There are no side-effects, only effects.

Businesses that really do get better at what they do can usually do more of it with fewer resources. They have competition to keep them on their toes. Their established services become cheaper and easier to deliver. Half their work doesn't involve patching up their earlier work. Behind the leading edge, their craft becomes more democratic, less centralised, much easier for the layperson to understand and access and apply on their own. Medicine seems to have become an exception to these rules.

Patrick Holford says people enter hospital 'horizontally ill', and leave 'vertically ill'[7]; meaning they get put back on their feet somehow, but not made well. Discharging you is the true unstated goal of any hospital department—whether home, perhaps with a lot of assistance, or into somebody else's department—not getting you healthy.

But true recovery is what takes place after the brilliant medical intervention, and must include overcoming the effects of the medical process itself.

State-run hospitals would give us the impression they are working only for the good of humanity, but they are still businesses, and must provide an income for legions of staff, administrators, service providers and suppliers. And if you leave still essentially unwell, you'll be back.

What gives some meaning to it all is the fact that many medical staff do care deeply about their patients and their work. They may strive to make life better for people. But the pharmaceutical mindset has them moving in the wrong direction, and they are obliged to follow it, or they are out.

Medical treatment alone seldom deals with why a diseased tissue became diseased in the first place. For example, one possible reason why so many cancers come back after surgery is that the tumour is merely a manifestation of a more general disease state in the patient. Removing the tumour is not the same as removing the cancer. Hence, chemotherapy is often included to poison the returning tumours and remaining cancer cells. But the problem is, it also poisons the patient. And since cancer is fundamentally a toxic state, the possible ramifications of further poisoning should be obvious.

Certainly, emergency care can sometimes give you back your life, but only you can restore your health. Emergency care can still make matters plenty worse, and it's vital to have your wits about you or good people on your side.

So, if there is any true health benefit to being in hospital, then it most likely comes from good nursing and a chance to rest. It certainly doesn't come from the hospital kitchen. The bottom line is you aren't likely to leave the hospital any healthier than you arrived.

Like long-life light bulbs and appliances that don't wear out, cures for disease are not good for business. They are painstaking and labour-intensive and can't be bottled or centralised. They involve washing faces and chopping vegetables and sourcing vitamins and giving sips of water and moving limbs around and walking people out into the garden and waiting—lots of waiting—and they don't fly practitioners around the world to glitzy conferences.

The practitioners and physicians who really solve these problems and also become very well-off are rare, and often get their real income from some other career, or with peripherals, such as retreats, room hire, teaching, or writing books.

And for every famous doctor or natural healer getting real results in terms of actual health, there must be literally thousands of unknown ones with holes in their shoes. Why? Because they are the ones with the knowledge, confidence, and ethical backbone to say, "Just wait a month."

Natural therapies, the ones that have been allowed to persist, are far from immune to these problems. I have worked in places where performance was gauged mainly on how patients felt after thirty minutes, or how many times you could get them to come back. Up-selling was encouraged. With such priorities, it is possible for almost any therapy to make a problem worse, insidiously. The clues tend to be more subtle than severe drug reactions or death on an operating table. They can be seen in therapy dependence; the perception of benefit but without a true reduction in need.

Most practitioners, and doctors even, will believe with utter sincerity that, even when there is ongoing unexplained degeneration, the therapy does wonders. It's just that the only answer to this particular patient's problems will be indefinite therapy. Sometimes it's true, but not always. The patient, in turn, will often believe that the therapy is "so good for me that I need it all the time to keep me going." They come away from a session with that 'Chinese Meal' effect, of feeling full to begin with but needing another meal very soon. Perhaps after a few more sessions, they will have some kind of 'breakthrough'. But the breakthroughs seldom happen, and the immense relief they got in the early stages of treatment becomes dulled with repeating therapy.

The term for this is palliation—making the patient feel better, or reducing the signs of their illness, but not really getting to grips with their problem. It is rife in the healing business, not least in medicine. The patient trying to find a real solution often has to traverse a minefield of well-meant palliation.

There are stories of celebrated practitioners having to move house when they retire: yet still their patients track them down, because they are hooked on the therapy that seems to help them so much that they simply can't get past always needing it.

I have had new patients come to me after decades of treatment with some highly respected therapists, bringing huge medication lists and with terribly complex problems. They insist that I just crack their back one more time because "it always worked when the last guy did it." Clearly it hadn't worked, and one look confirms that more of the same is not what they need. They can leave disappointed and even angry when told that what they are asking is dangerous, or that a fresh start is now needed.

Health means, above all else, independence. This progression towards dependence on therapies is not healthy. And, whether through medical or alternative treatment, it arises from a few things: treating effects not causes, ignoring guiding principles, looking too narrowly at the problem, or going at it in too direct or linear a way.

Put another way, it comes from failing to recognise the truly slippery nature of complex systems such as living humans. It may be sold as holistic, but, natural or not, it is the antithesis of holism. Dealing with complexity is what holism is all about, and I will explore that throughout the book.

Few healers set out to be less than the best. As much as anything, the abundance of impressive quick fixes comes as a result of what survives in the marketplace. Renowned skill and quick relief bring people into your business, but once they get better, they fire you. Bravura palliation can convey an impression of mastery and keep the patient coming back for years. The moral is, know your stuff but don't think too deeply.

I'm not going to say much more about palliation, except that any therapy can be used in a palliative way.

It doesn't need to be like this, and I don't believe it always was. There seems to have been a great wave of natural healers during the 18th and 19th centuries, and there is a lot that they knew, both about keeping well and restoring health, that has been forgotten or actively taken away.

When faced with illness in 1850, hundreds of miles from a hospital, what do you do? Is it better to load up the wagon and hope you survive the journey? Or deal with it at home? Should you take the risks of decisive action? Or leave things alone and pray? You don't have all the ideal tools and knowledge, so how do you use the resources that you have?

Without drug stores on every corner, healers in the wild west of America needed a set of fundamental principles to guide them. They relied on an approach that was part scientific, part philosophical; and an understanding of nature's laws. Then they set to work with whatever they had to hand.

As knowledge improved and reliable drugs appeared— and railways, and towns, and hospitals in the towns—the resources available to the sick increased. Solutions that got you back to work quickest also got your attention. Nuanced, in-depth consideration of the problem wasn't always a winner when there was a harvest to bring in.

Eventually, along came antibiotics and other magic bullets. It was no longer necessary to look to patterns in nature, to help guess which item from the kitchen cupboard to try first. Just take the pill and things will improve, for the moment. That is, until the antibiotics didn't work, or it turned out that those other magic bullets were causing problems. But by then, the trajectory was set. Chemical medicine had staked its claim as the rational way forward. More chemistry, better magic bullets, was the answer. The old guy harping on about nature's laws didn't hold much sway in the big corporate hospital. Get the patient on his feet and out. Get the lab people onto it. Get the government to pay them. Why not?

It is only when the magic bullets run out of power that we get a sense of something missing from this dazzling cornucopia of brilliant technical fixes.

And I will argue that medicine has gone so far down the magic bullet route that it is causing more problems than it is solving—that we need a set of guiding principles more than ever. Moreover, that when we rediscover those healing principles, we can manage without much of the rocket science. When we do occasionally need the hospital, we could engage with it more judiciously. We would know what questions to ask. The hospital would understand our needs better.

These fundamental guiding principles are what I mean by missing links.

And back then there was also a great deal of dross, old wives' tales, and dangerous quackery, which did cause harm, and made it easy to justify the land grab. Once again, a baseline of fundamental principles could help us sort the wheat from the chaff.

With a bit of education and a return of some old ideas, we don't need 'nannying' by the medical system, we just need a chance to pursue our own destiny. As it is structured, medicine does not allow that. As a patient, I wouldn't dream of telling a doctor or surgeon how to do his job; all I ask for is an informed and truly free choice on whether to take him up on his offer.

Other missing links are the concepts that may have been employed unconsciously by good practitioners for centuries, that were perhaps unstated, waiting for the right language to encapsulate them. They have already shown their worth, but still go unrecognised as concepts. They may be the mysterious magic which seems to exist by special intuition in the hands of certain talented therapists. All that is needed to share them is the right lexicon, and an open mind to accept their value.

Then there are the *missing links* yet to be discovered, and I don't claim to offer anything new. If all I can do is make some overlooked ideas more accessible, then I will be satisfied.

And of course, there are the 'latest things' ... and generally, I am cautious of those for two reasons. For one, that the 'latest things' often turn out to be duds at best or harmful at worst. And for another, that they are simply not needed. If the means to maintain and restore health were not within us, we would already be dead.

If you are waiting for a medical breakthrough to save you, prepare for disappointment. The history of medical innovation is littered with false promises and deadly mistakes. Ideas that prove worthy in healing are generally favoured by maturity and experience, not by novelty. They are also favoured by having a clear framework of understanding, as much as an impressive repertoire of methods.

So, the following is a collection of essays on how healers of all kinds may avoid the many shortcuts typical of medicine but not exclusive to medicine, in order to be more effective. This is also to avoid sowing the seeds of more complex disease later, and ultimately, of long, drawn-out, unpleasant ends in our lives, as well.

For that reason, I have added a final section on what is the ultimate medical shortcut, something euphemistically called pathways.

The ethics in that subject have become muddled, but the hope is to avoid having to face that dilemma at all, if possible. I know which side of the fence I am on. I don't believe it is the job of a healer to end life, and I am firm with that. The trouble is, that all healers, not just doctors, risk-taking shortcuts, knowingly or otherwise, that might eventually contribute to those sorts of dilemmas.

There is a lot of overlap between the chapters. You will see the same themes repeated several times from different perspectives, and that is intentional, since it is necessary to see how these links work together as a chain. It also means the whole should be visible within any of the parts. The challenge of making it all digestible has been enormous, and this short work pops out after many years of gestation.

This book has been written from the perspective of an osteopath who left the profession after I realised it had drifted far off course long before I took up the discipline. I didn't get into this business for a title: I did it to solve a difficult problem in my own life. And now that I have solved it, the title seems irrelevant, and it's time for the next set of challenges. I do not claim to speak for the profession I have left or those who remain part of it.

Importantly, osteopathy doesn't have a monopoly on any technique or idea, and the intention is that much of this can be exported to any other field of healing. This isn't about how to do things, but how to think about the things we do.

So, if you want to learn some long-forgotten osteopathic technique for stomach ulcers, you'll be disappointed. But if you want to know how an osteopath, 100 years ago, might have thought about a stomach ulcer, then just expand on any or all of the principles herein.

Importantly, I don't claim to treat ulcers or anything else with a medical name, not even back pain. Names for conditions can be unhelpful and misleading, except occasionally as a starting point for investigation. Once again, health is the only solution to disease, and it doesn't work selectively. A true health discipline works universally, and can be applied to anything, more or less, short of near-death emergencies.

I'm going to warn you in advance ... I do bash medicine quite a lot. It is quite clear that medicine has a lot to answer for, so I am not ashamed of this. This is not to put down the many very decent people working in medicine, or to lose sight of the good that medicine can still do, but rather to explain why we urgently need something better, and to paint a background against which to see these other ideas more clearly.

I also raise issues with certain therapies, and again, it is mainly for the purpose of contrast. I have only mentioned those with which I have some familiarity. All have something to offer, and all have imperfections. What

matters most when choosing a therapy is the vision of
the individual practitioner, not what flag they fly.

That said, most therapies are positively defined by
their methods, and one or two are defined by conditions,
or by certain anatomical regions or systems. In my view,
these are in-built flaws that most will struggle to overcome, since the selectivity baked into those definitions
works counter to the idea of health as a general state.

What should define us as therapists is how we think
about our patient's situation, and the process of inferring
treatment from that. Osteopathy does not mean rubbing
muscles and treating back pain. Osteopathy means gross
physiology, and that is as good a definition as any.

And I also touch on politics, because if anything in life
is political, it is healthcare. One of the most obvious ways
central control creeps in to affect the patient-practitioner
relationship is through regulation, and my position now is
that I no longer see much benefit in healthcare regulation.
If there really were free choice in healthcare, then regulation would not be needed, since there is nothing it can
do that market forces, free-speech, and pre-existing con-
sumer protections can't do much better. We already have
the right not to be harmed, killed, or defrauded by our
doctors. As a patient myself, I no longer feel protected by
regulation—quite the reverse, as I will explain in stages.
For starters, regulation has become part of a direct line
from government policy straight through to the patient,
and that isn't good.

Then there is this Jekyll and Hyde duality called Public
Health. What was once a respectable way to ensure good
living conditions has morphed into a system for imposing

government policy and blanket medication on the unwilling masses. In recent times, it has been seen coming at its victims with harsh dictates and medical mandates before disappearing, shapeless and unidentified into the fog.

As holists, we must remain holistic at all times. Partly holistic is an oxymoron. We talk about treating the whole person, invoking the body's own healing mechanisms and working with nature; avoiding drugs and quick fixes. But what do these things mean? And how do we avoid the trap of doing just the opposite? Sorting out these things means beginning with a clear idea of what a complete healing system looks like.

Long before I was a practitioner, I was a patient. And this is also a book for the patient, about how to understand your own healing journey; whether or not you are currently looking for treatment. I hope to offer you a better chance of recognising what is going on, navigating your situation well, identifying valid help and avoiding the duds, and ultimately finding the independence that is the universal defining feature of health.

[1] Li L, Geraghty OC, Mehta Z, Rothwell PM; Oxford Vascular Study. *Age-specific risks, severity, time course, and outcome of bleeding on long-term antiplatelet treatment after vascular events: a population-based cohort study.* The Lancet. 2017 Jul 29;390(10093):490-499. doi: 10.1016/S0140-6736(17)30770-5. Epub 2017 Jun 13. PMID: 28622955; PMCID: PMC5537194.

[2] Dan Jones, *Darwinian medicine: Does intensive care kill or cure?* New Scientist, 11 Aug 2010.

https://www.newscientist.com/article/mg20727731-600-darwinian-medicine-does-intensive-care-kill-or-cure/.

[3] Cunningham SA, Mitchell K, Narayan KM, Yusuf S. *Doctors' strikes and mortality: a review.* Soc Sci Med. 2008 Dec;67(11):1784-8. doi: 10.1016/j.socscimed.2008.09.044. Epub 2008 Oct 10. PMID: 18849101.

[4] *Fewer paramedics means more lives saved*, Firefighter Close Calls, https://www.firefighterclosecalls.com/fewer-paramedics-means-more-lives-saved/.

[5] A Midwestern Doctor, *The monopolization of medicine*, https://www.midwesterndoctor.com/p/dermatologys-disastrous-war-against.

[6] *US Judge Finds Medical Group Conspired Against Chiropractors*, New York Times, 29 Aug 1987, https://www.nytimes.com/1987/08/29/us/us-judge-finds-medical-group-conspired-against-chiropractors.html.

[7] Patrick Holford, book, *The Optimum Nutrition Bible.*

Natural medicine, or 'medicine lite'?

*Being honest may not get you a lot of friends
but it'll always get you the right ones.*

—attributed to John Lennon

The natural hygienists of the 19th century, the early osteopaths, and homoeopaths, had far better ideas about how to engage with complex living systems than modern medicine, a statement I will justify in due course. And they drew upon ideas that go back at least as far as Hippocrates.

The drift into pharmaceutical dominance became a coordinated land grab in around 1910, when the Carnegie Foundation commissioned Abraham Flexner to perform a survey of medical training in the United States. Outwardly, the intention was to raise standards and bring medicine into the scientific age. But the effect was to promote pharmacy-based approaches to medicine, and to suppress any kind of nature cure. More than half the schools in America closed down; some because of poor standards of course, but also those that could not or would not conform to the expected paradigms.

After that, a huge amount of financial assistance was poured into medical training, much of it by the Rockefeller Foundation, in order to buy influence over the training [1].

New language and thinking tools emerged, and it is now very hard to escape them, even when supposedly engaged in alternative medical practice.

These changes were designed to take our attention away from what we really need for health and place the emphasis on bottled products. Why deal with the thorny issues of a stressful and toxic existence when you can just take a pill instead? Better still, why even think about those things, since the pill is the only real treatment, anyway? And in a way, our training and cultural indoctrination have turned the pill into the only treatment with any real power, as I'll explain.

An alternative therapy doesn't mean treating a medical diagnosis with a leaf instead of a drug. The drug probably came from the leaf, in any case. What it means is having an alternative framework for understanding the patient's situation, and from that, inferring the best way to help. If we take away the framework of understanding, the method loses its potency.

In the wake of the Flexner Report, a lot of truly powerful knowledge was lost, much of it very low tech and hard to centralise. The changes inevitably spread throughout the world, so that doctors in one country now speak very much the same language as in any other. Some therapies survived by denying their true faith. The osteopaths in the United States, for instance, have become prescribers, and all but a few work in a disease-based model.

This inevitably leads to direct or linear therapy (terms I'll explain later), and those who don't toe the line can find it difficult to get ahead.

The chiropractors resisted these changes to an extent, or more exactly, stood their ground against the power grab that ensued. They are to be admired for their legal and political savvy. But since theirs is inherently a very direct therapy, I am not sure how much philosophical ground they managed to hold, if any.

The final nail in the coffin for osteopathy in the UK was the pursuit of regulation, and in order to offer training, the colleges had to dovetail their curricula with regulatory frameworks. And that meant that the clinical side at least had to be consistent with medical standards.

Osteopathic patient assessment now largely consists of orthopaedic and neurological examination, specific tissue diagnosis, and pathology screening, with the aim of weeding out anything 'medical' or 'systemic'. This leads absolutely anywhere but holistic care, and hopefully later you will see the difference, if you don't already know.

Osteopaths will say they are considering 'osteopathic principles'. But how can they be, when the very reasoning process they have drummed into them assumes medical divisions within the body, and medical classifications for diseases? We make it seem better by kidding ourselves there is no philosophy, only truth, and science. But in coming chapters, I will show that this is inadequate.

Even when osteopaths do drift cautiously into the 'functional' or 'systemic', they do so in a highly modular manner, drawing on other 'modalities' for those aspects. This very framework sets them up as adjunctive to medicine and not alternative. The thanks they receive for playing the game is that the profession has, if anything, been attacked even harder for any perceived shortcoming, and at times it seems no argument is good enough for the critics.

This is not alternative medicine: it is the esoteric application of conventional medicine. And it is made to work by leaving out the square pegs that won't fit into those round holes. And thus, a limited scope of practice has emerged.

As a practitioner, you can still have any ideas you want, as long as you practise them lawfully and ethically. But in order to use a protected title, you first have to spend several gruelling years making all the right noises in a government approved institution. The chances of coming through this brainwashing with your world view unadjusted are slim. And if you do, you will face so much professional difficulty that you will sooner or later have to make compromises, anyway.

Thus, regulated therapists must base their interventions on a foundation of medical theory, more or less, directly. In Australia and New Zealand, it is even worse, since regulated practitioners can be audited, which includes reviewing confidential records even without the consent of the patient. Many patients receive government funding for their treatment, and in New Zealand, practitioners' notes are checked, at random, by the administrators at Accident Compensation Corporation (ACC) to see if they agree with the assessment. If they do not, then the practitioner—the one who actually got the patient better—will be asked to adjust their approach.

And guess whose standards will be applied in the check-ing process? Not the patient, who knows better than anybody, whether or not they benefited. And not even the practitioner, the one who actually spends all day with real patients, and perhaps saw something crucial in the case that those administrators wouldn't even recognise as valid.

What this all means for the practitioner is a sense of somebody breathing down their neck. In turn, the patient can never fully trust that the practitioner is working for them. The administrative classes thrive on these arrange-ments and are not likely to want it all reversed.

To date, the system has, in effect, manufactured a divide between patient and practitioner, and thus con-trived a need for the protection it is there to provide. At the same time, it is setting up conditions where the most dangerous kinds of healthcare possible—those based on poisons—get elevated. Even those who have stayed out of the regulated fields have not escaped these influences.

In removing the truly holistic, health-based, and patient-centred theories of the natural healers of old, the Flexner Report and the reforms that followed have stifled competition and held medicine back 100 years.

For all the massive resources, powerful technology and up-to-the-minute science available to the modern doc-tor, medicine's engagement with the patient is positively medieval. In essence, it is still driving out disease in the belief that health will thereby remain behind. And you can see it in the hospitals. They are not fit places for the pursuit of health. If they were, then people would want to visit them often and stay as long as possible. You're lucky if there is a window you can open. If a healthy person went there for a month, he might easily end up sick.

In modern times, some practitioners became aware of something missing and, wanting better for their patients, went looking to find it. With such imposed conceptual limitations, they naturally went in search of more tools. Growth in courses for practitioners has been huge, and they almost entirely revolve around the idea of 'modalities'; that is to say … ways of delivering treatment. Modalities are good for business, but reflecting on where we are going with it all doesn't necessarily pay the bills.

The result is that there are now almost limitless courses in techniques of every kind, but very few on what it is we are actually trying to do with them. Some healers will even refuse to discuss guiding principles of any kind, parroting such nonsense, as it is wrong to impose our own thinking upon the patient, as if the patient were somehow a prisoner. Having a clear set of guiding principles and sticking to them is not imposition, it is competence. Yet when it is suggested to those same practitioners that they don't stand for anything, they can get very defensive.

If you want to see imposed thinking in action, just visit any hospital.

What the new breed of post-war natural therapists achieved was mainly to fill up their toolboxes with a greater variety of tools, rather than unearthing any hidden blueprint for health. Hence, we still have all the ingredients for a great cake; it is the recipe that is now missing.

The chiropractors developed into a fine art the skills of adjusting every bone in many different ways. But the thinking process appears still wholly medical: identify a quasi-pathological cause and neutralise it head-on with a specific correction. They had been allowed the freedom to sell their undoubtedly brilliant techniques, but to do what?

In my own field of osteopathy, practitioners wanting more than expertise in sore backs, branched out into other areas, such as herbs and needling, and developed new methods, like stretching fascia or working with the ebb and flow of the fluids of the body, sometimes known as the cranial rhythm. They learned how to adjust the organs and nerves directly with their hands. Lots more new and exciting ingredients came, but still no recipe.

And so it was that, in the quest for renewed acceptance, the homoeopaths pitched their energetic remedies against drugs, inevitably testing specific remedies against specific conditions in a pretty standard research model. Osteopaths entertained demands to test spinal manipulation for back pain, as if that were synonymous with testing osteopathy for health. It isn't the same at all. Tailoring homoeopathic remedies to the constitution (discussed later), as they are meant to be prescribed, gets people better, but it defies standard research methods more appropriate for drugs. Thus, entering an effective natural therapy into clinical research usually sets it up to fail.

Consider this: performing a randomised trial on a bespoke therapy makes no more sense than doing a randomised trial on tailor-made suits. Your trial will only prove that tailor-made suits don't fit, and that randomly pulling suits off shelves in Marks and Spencer works just as well.

Still, trials of techniques against medical conditions did produce tantalising nuggets of evidence. Frustratingly, they also cast a great deal of doubt on the potency many patients and practitioners had witnessed personally, and played into the hands of a whole industry of scepticism. Few could see the problem with the style of research, and many felt that if it was good enough for drugs, it ought to be good enough for other therapies.

What was being overlooked was the relentless sleight of hand being employed in the testing of drugs. The same methodologies and flawed reasoning that are used to make drugs look better have also made natural therapies look worse. Thus, a lot of good ideas got discarded and bad ones adopted as the mainstream. The categorisations and hierarchies that follow are unreasonable.

These explorations in reductionist territory did certainly bear some fruit. Developing modalities and new skills to fill the void, where once a great richness of theory and philosophy had been, produced good enough results to keep natural healers in business, but not so good as to compete with medicine on medicine's terms.

It all cemented the direction for development ever since, shaping natural medicine as a sort of 'medicine lite': reasonably useful for mild conditions but not powerful enough for the big stuff.

And, if any natural healer dares to go for 'the big stuff', like cancer, he risks punishment, even if his solutions turn out to be 100% effective: worse still, if he advises against the standard medical offerings. The UK's 1939 Cancer Act and worldwide equivalent measures make sure of it. Anti-competitive practices don't come any more blatant than pulling strings to write laws against the competition. Medicine lite is how natural medicine is now viewed almost universally.

The thing is, there is no natural law to say that the difficulty of solving a problem is proportional to the severity of its effects. Scurvy, for example, is a life-threatening condition with severe symptoms that is not hard to prevent or reverse: all it takes is a mindset to recognise it.

Some doctors believe scurvy is coming back. Given how useful Vitamin C is as a therapeutic, I'm not convinced it ever really went away. And where is the will to do something about it? The last time I took vitamins to someone in hospital, they got locked in a cupboard and I had to protest strongly to get them back. A fair assessment of the varying degrees in which scurvy persists in the population, often misdiagnosed, might render many medical treatments redundant and give power back to the people [2]. This is just one example of why medicine might need to keep a grip on the competition, even if the cost is the truth about human health.

Yet we have arrived at a place where, openly, non-medical practitioners can only treat 'mild' conditions in those who are not deemed 'pathological'. More severe conditions, and cases that don't respond on those same terms, are to be handed over to 'real' doctors, who very often are just as stumped as anybody else.

For my antidote to the problem, read on.

[1] Stahnisch FW, Verhoef M. *The Flexner Report of 1910 and its impact on complementary and alternative medicine and psychiatry in north America in the 20th century. Evid Based Complement Alternat Med.*

2012;2012:647896. doi: 10.1155/2012/647896. Epub 2012 Dec 26. PMID: 23346209; PMCID: PMC3543812.

[2] Sydney Morning Herald, *Scurvy surprise: Archaic sickness that struck down sailors resurfaces in Sydney,* 29 Nov 2016, https://www.smh.com.au/healthcare/scurvy-surprise-archaic-sickness-that-struck-down-sailors-resurfaces-in-sydney-20161129-gszrhx.html.

Notes on evidence and referencing

If we lose all the universities, then we would lose nothing.
But if we lose the forests, we lose everything.

—Bill Mollison

This is a work about important principles and patterns, not an encyclopaedia of isolated facts. I have suggested some further reading here and there. Anyone is welcome to explore these hypotheses in their own way, improve them or find better ideas, and I would urge the reader to do that.

What I don't advocate is experimentation on patients or misrepresenting the degree of certainty in clinical treatment. What can be inferred from here in terms of therapeutic methods is down to what the individual practitioner infers from it. Step one in employing these ideas is simply to carry on business as usual, and see if you can spot the same patterns.

Initially, I did think to fill these pages with references and citations, but too many citations can be misleading or even steer the narrative. The trouble is that research and industry are like the white and yolk of a scrambled egg—we can't just unscramble them. To sort things out, we need some fresh material.

Besides, my overall position is a summation of what I have gathered over several decades and leans only lightly on formal data. Try as I might, it may be hard to find or even remember the original sources. But the lessons learned have endured. At times, the source might only be something I heard in a college lecture, a conversation with a colleague, a nugget from a patient, or something I have pieced together from experience. Every argument one ever makes has holes, and sometimes they let in more light. There will be errors, but they are made in good faith, and I hope they aren't sufficient to ruin the overall picture.

It is common in medicine and science to be asked for evidence, to tie all one's thinking to theories that have been accepted by peers, as if that proves a solid foundation.

The reality is that medicine still invokes many unproven ideas, many superstitions, and some quite cuckoo notions that have never been proven. Ice for an ankle sprain is one obvious example. Staying away from salt and butter to avoid heart disease is another. The biggest whopper of them all is that we need poisons to keep ourselves healthy … and that one is baked right through the cake.

There is also plenty of narrative where the research seems tight but has underpinnings that are unproven nonsense. Later on I'll cover some examples. And in case anybody still believes in the infallibility of scientists, the most searched and cited scientific paper of all time is the one by John Ioannidis—*Why Most Published Research*

Findings Are False [1]. Without meaning to be flippant, no, I haven't read the whole paper.

Moreover, denial of the unusual or the unorthodox stifles excellence. This might be okay if standardisation led to better outcomes overall. Just as likely, it sets up the same mediocrity everywhere. Calling it 'best practice' is a play on words.

Formal practice is supposed to be guided by what is called the *best available evidence*. There is a hierarchy to help us choose, with the randomised controlled trial (RCT) somewhere near the top, and anecdotal observation somewhere near the bottom. Newer studies are supposed to carry more weight than older ones. The best evidence of all is supposed to be the *meta-analysis*, in which as many valid studies as possible are pooled together.

This academic construct spills over into commentary and discussion of every kind. But it is obviously flawed, and later I will discuss some very real problems with evidence-based medicine generally.

Quite simply, the best available evidence is the evidence that is most relevant.

By that I mean that a single anecdote can sometimes save the day, in a situation where the entire back catalogue of The Lancet has nothing useful to offer.

So, which is the best evidence—anecdote, RCT or meta-analysis? The answer is, whichever one provides the most helpful insight into your problem. This cannot be determined before the fact by committees of academics.

The zeal for solid evidence is a way to marginalise some of the most important knowledge available, that born of experience, insight, intuition, pattern recognition or serendipity. There is a purpose to such marginalisation, and the purpose is control. Medical products are heavily marketed, and tight control of narratives serves that purpose. Institutions do need to have some unity of message or else things will fall apart. In the case of medicine, such unity comes at the price of the doctor's independent judgement.

On the other hand, the demand for evidence also has a laudable purpose, and that is accountability. Nobody should do anything in medicine that can't be justified. Unfortunately, justifying decisions is a far cry from improving outcomes, and many medical decisions plainly protect the doctor more than the patient. Justification is an imprecise idea, and it has to take into account many human, scientific, and practical considerations. Summing it all up algorithmically as *true or false* isn't good enough.

Nevertheless, there is nothing new under the sun, and I don't claim to offer any new ideas. Everything in this book is attached to things I have been taught or read elsewhere, or actually observed. I have seen it compared with real life and it compares very well. I am not an academic by any means. I came into healing with a knowledge of spanners, and engines, and getting hurt falling out of aeroplanes, and eventually having a sick relative in hospital—real world stuff—not from reading books about cells and molecules. Hence, I don't have much time for academics who say that the bumblebee isn't mathematically capable of flight.

"They have an answer for everything, but if it were a bridge they were building, it would fall down," my sister once said after a meeting with hospital consultants.

I have forgotten where I learned much of this, but I have seen it fit the facts in other people's practice and my own, and in the countless stories people have told me about their own healing journeys. It's just that some of the origins have been lost. I have adopted these ideas because the mainstream of healing that I once believed was the absolute pinnacle of reason has shown itself to be riddled with problems.

I am not alone in taking a minimal approach to referencing. One core text, practically our college bible on physiology, had not one single reference [2]. What it did contain was a list of expert contributors. In other words, it was entirely a work of opinion. Where those contributors got their beliefs from is not clear, and their sources could have been anything from solid research right down to "that is our best guess." This would be excusable, except for one thing. A huge amount of vitally important medical science rests on that sort of foundation, claiming to be absolutely solid, while overlooking valid competing theories.

Therefore, as a backstop, we need reservoirs of ideas for when our reservoirs of facts turn out to be polluted. At the risk of ridicule, this book is my contribution. It is meant as a useful sketch of a huge problem and its solution, and not as a watertight case. I have included some references for background information, especially where the claims are controversial or startling. But the substantive ideas are my distillation. The proof is somewhere out there, or most of it.

Let us not lose sight of the value that exists in experience, tradition, knowledge passed person-to-person, and best guesses.

I once had a maths teacher who said, "Put down your pens; if you're taking notes, you're not thinking." So please leave your textbooks on the shelf and turn off your internet. Save the fact checking for later.

I want you to grasp the narrative, otherwise you will miss the point and won't know which facts to check. The ideas presented here are at times subtle and at times quite meaty. But they may be unfamiliar and, therefore, may take time to process. Do your own research, but please do it afterwards.

[1] Ioannidis JPA (2005) *Why Most Published Research Findings Are False*. PLOS Medicine 2(8): e124. https://doi.org/10.1371/journal.pmed.0020124.

[2] *Principles of anatomy and physiology*, ninth edition, Gerard J. Tortora, Sandra R. Grabowski.

Missing Link 1: How we measure success

Torture numbers and they'll confess to anything.

—Gregg Easterbrook, writer and journalist

Natural therapists will debate passionately about whether something works or not, or whether one approach works better than the other. When comparisons with medical treatment are brought into it, the debate gets truly political: and it's unsurprising when we consider how much money is at stake. At that level, people lose jobs for holding the wrong opinions about what works. There is an entire industry devoted to making pharmaceuticals look good under the guise of objective and impartial research, and suppressing opposition; and all supposedly in the name of protecting the public.

For example, did you know that Borax was declared a poison soon after it was found that traces can safely and significantly relieve arthritis? Arthritis is big business, and something to rival it that costs pennies a year is a threat to a huge and well-connected industry.

The degree to which pharmaceuticals control information and legislation cannot be overestimated. Drug company Pfizer alone spends in the region of $2bn a year on advertising [1]. That's quite remarkable, since only two countries in the world—New Zealand and the USA—permit direct television advertising of drugs. Hence, much effort surely has to be directed creatively into other ways to promote their message. Indirect pharmaceutical marketing through scientific publishing, education, medical law and regulation, and ongoing professional development for medical practitioners, means the true total can't easily be reckoned. It's hard to imagine that there wouldn't be considerable editorial control in news, television, journals and social media, all of which benefit from drug company money one way or another.

Direct medical interests show up three times in the top ten lobby groups of the American government [2]. The second biggest donor to the World Health Organisation, after the government of the USA, is the Bill and Melinda Gates Foundation, which also has a colossal stake in the vaccine industry [3]. There can be little doubt that private enterprise gathers considerable influence through such arrangements. And to what end?

The other side of this is that bashing alternative medicine is a business in itself. Yes, really. In 1987, a federal court in the USA found the American Medical Association (AMA) guilty of conspiring to destroy chiropractic [4]. The court ordered the AMA to dismantle the operation, but this follows a pattern of behaviour going back many years, and some claim the function was handed over to others to continue. There may be undisclosed private interests behind the recent 'skeptics' movement and so-called 'fact-checking' industries [5]. Wikipedia editing in certain subject areas seems highly coordinated [6].

What I find alarming is that it is so much harder even to gather information about all this than it was even a few years ago. It used to be far more transparent. But now, search engines are unashamedly part of the crusade against so-called 'disinformation and misinformation', which in reality means anything they don't want you to know.

The Advertising Standards Authority (ASA) in the UK has a systemic bias against anything non-medical, since it maintains narrow lists of 'conditions' that alternative practitioners can mention in advertising. This emphasis on conditions is a trap if we rise to it. Their one and only criterion seems to be what is shown in published randomised controlled trials, a system that big pharma games with ease. At the very least, it appears that the administrators at the ASA, who lack our training, have a crude understanding of clinical practice in some fields. Who advises them, and for what reason, might be another issue.

Whatever really lurks behind the private enterprise known as advertising standards, this raises a broader issue about how the question of effectiveness is considered.

That's all an aside, or would be, if we could rest assured that our perceptions of what is safe and effective were not being quite heavily adjusted.

Much of the heat could be removed from the effectiveness argument by clearing up what exactly we mean by saying something works. It's wrong to say Borax 'works' for arthritis, because Borax doesn't cure or treat anything. It's that traces of Boron, the essential element in Borax, are a requirement of life and health. Many cases of arthritis, osteoporosis, and other things may be a result of its deficiency. To call it a cure for arthritis is as nonsensical as saying water is a cure for dehydration. Insufficiencies in our basic needs should never be medicalised, but they are. Incidentally, I don't recommend taking Borax, since its illegality as a food item means that one can't be sure of the purity. Better to get an actual Boron supplement.

Practitioners and physicians will often end an argument by saying, "Well, it works." What do they mean? Does it relieve symptoms? Causes? How fast? For a short while or for all time? For everybody or a few? At a cost to overall health? And so on.

It is no good saying the patient felt better after treatment if one fails to mention that terminal cancer could be a consequence. And yet, that is in the profile of steroid drugs. On the one hand, something works if there is relief from inflammation, or the patient can breathe again. And so, steroids certainly have their uses. On the other hand, it doesn't work if it kills the patient. But a steroid medication can do both, to the same patient. So, does it work, or not? We can see the need for nuance. But when a practitioner says their technique 'works', it is nuance they are hoping to avoid.

Natural therapies can do it as well. Spinal manipulation, for instance, can relieve back pain very quickly in some cases, leading patients with even mild symptoms to describe their osteopath as a genius. Used in too direct a way, it can also lead to a destabilisation of the posture, resulting in plenty of repeat business for years to come, until the underlying degeneration gets so severe that no amount of isolated cracking relieves the pain.

At that point, the patient may be on medication, not just for the back pain, but for other acquired health problems that are easily not associated with it in the minds of anyone involved. These progressions contain an in-built deniability, in the same way that no sufferer of inflammatory bowel disease can prove it was their drugs that caused them cancer.

And even as they harbour deeply entrenched postural disturbance and long medication lists after twenty years of cracking, the patient will be as loyal to their genius practitioner as ever. It doesn't have to be like that when manipulation is used in the right way. But without some framework to discuss these issues, we have no way to get ahead with this. The framework begins with being clear on what we mean when we say something works.

Extending the back pain example, we easily forget that back pain is not a condition. It is a *symptom*, with a million possible causes. We can use the same techniques to address the causes or to address the symptoms, or both, depending on our blueprint for their use: but the long-term effects over time will be vastly divergent.

Hypothetically at least, one therapist will help you be well, the other, however, could make you sick eventually, using the same techniques, and you can't possibly know after the first few sessions.

The chances of the practitioner being able to explain the difference are remote. Whenever I asked in college why we were learning to crack joints, the result was often an embarrassed silence. No truly deep and coherent answer ever came. It was generally accepted within the college community that it could have deeper physiological effects, but there was a distinct lack of structured guidance on how to apply it to that end.

The teaching was by no means sloppy: in fact, academic rigour was the college's forte. It's just that this is a notoriously difficult discussion.

"It relieves pain and increases mobility," was the safe answer. "It works," in other words.

It took me a very long time to get to grips with the question properly, since even the most expert 'back crackers' I knew couldn't articulate a very clear explanation, if they had one. Yet spinal adjustment is potentially so much more.

I'm afraid I can't offer the answer here either, not because I don't have one, but because it would take a separate work to cover it properly. However, I will offer some background concepts in the later chapters on complexity, patterns, and gravity. Understanding those should be the starting point.

One way drug therapies get around the question of effectiveness is by narrowing down the outcome measures, and it seems natural therapists aren't slow to do the same thing. It goes something like this. Research finds that the drug reduces heart attacks: sounds good so far. Then, buried in the report or obfuscated by jargon: over the few months' duration of the trial, in certain carefully selected groups of people, as long as we gave it to a large enough number, and they mustn't eat grapefruit. Truly: if you are prescribed statins you are supposed to avoid grapefruit. And don't forget to mention that side-effects are few, as long as we give them an impressive enough name, like rhabdomyolysis (muscle break-down), or dementia. Because, after all, those are different diseases, and we're only interested in heart problems. But give us more money and we can do something for those as well.

Yes, it really is like that! Did you know there is a condition called 'Failed Back Surgery Syndrome' (FBSS)? Yes, seriously. There are whole departments devoted to FBSS. Your surgery went well: it was a new medical condition that crippled you. This perfectly illustrates why hospitals are getting bigger, not smaller.

Researchers will change their minds, anyway. Last year's medical textbook is this year's landfill.

Back to natural therapy: I wouldn't feel good if somebody's treatment for back pain 'worked' but six sessions later they develop acid reflux, headaches, or a heart disturbance. I would want to know what I had overlooked. The 'accepted' way to address this is to say the new problem is nothing to do with the back treatment: "Go and see your doctor for that and I'll treat you for your back."

This was the way we were taught to do it in college. But at that stage, we have no right to claim our therapy is holistic, and any practitioner who compartmentalises the body that way and claims to be a holist is, in my view, a fraud. And once one's eyes are open to what really makes natural healing different from medicine, it isn't good enough.

It would be hard these days to get the connection between spinal adjustment and general health taken seriously in any scientific or medical quarter. But it is the original reason, I believe, that osteopaths and chiropractors have to learn the physiology of the organs.

Another way drug therapies approach effectiveness is by what are called surrogate measures or markers. The reasoning goes like this: being overweight is associated with poor health. So, if we just make everybody thinner somehow, they will be healthier. But what matters is not the weight lost, but the change in health it signifies. You can lose weight with stomach surgery, or amphetamines, but that is a far cry from saying you are healthier. In fact, your life could be shortened by either approach.

Weight is an example of a surrogate measure for health. In some ways, we need such markers to determine where our patient is at. But if we look only at a single marker as a precise measure for success, then we miss the real targets by miles. In short, you don't get healthy by losing weight, but you might lose weight by getting healthy.

A person with high cholesterol or high blood pressure also has those things high because they need to be high. It's not to say they are ideal situations, it's just to say that weight, cholesterol, and blood pressure are *results* of our health, but not *drivers* of health, and, in isolation, they are poor markers for health as well. They could even be preventing catastrophic failure of some kind. More on that later.

On the other hand, if the homoeostatic regulation of these things has gone wrong, then it is the regulation that needs to be addressed, and not the endpoint.

The point is that having high blood pressure and high cholesterol is not synonymous with having heart disease. Therefore, as markers for heart disease, they are surrogates. Therapeutically speaking, *simply bringing the numbers up or down does not make a person healthy.*

It is one thing saying that high cholesterol signifies heart disease. It might, but that's a whole subject in itself [7]. The question we should be asking is whether simply suppressing the production of cholesterol with drugs will make matters any better. The answer is it doesn't. We need to get to grips with why the cholesterol is high. If somebody is overweight and has high blood pressure, we need to wonder why. And on all those subjects, we have been fed wrong answers our entire lives.

The moral is, trust your body: it knows what it is doing. And if you don't believe that, then don't be a healer.

One of the most misleading surrogate measures of all is in the vaccination programme. Politicians love to say that putting pressure on parents to vaccinate their children has been a big public health success.

"Look," they say, "we now have far more children vaccinated than ever." Big deal. Empty syringes don't, by any stretch, mean healthier children, but they would like us to think so. Their claims that this has been successful are meaningless without some accompanying data on the health of those children.

The big questions that follow then, are: what really is health, how do we define it if not by sets of numbers, and how do we achieve it?

The way to assess properly what 'works' is to broaden out the outcome measures as much as possible, and to look at all areas of health, for the lifetime of the patient. Once we understand, for instance, that back pain is a symptom, not a problem, then what matters is not that the patient is less achy after a few minutes. It is how much independence they regain, how long they live, how few drugs they are on, or what other problems they develop, avoid, or overcome through treatment.

I'm always delighted, of course, when the patient says they are feeling better at the end of the session. But just as many have a rocky ride to begin with before they really get back their freedom within their own bodies. If they are sore for a while, it's not that the therapy has hurt them, or shouldn't be. It's that the healing process itself can invoke symptoms of its own, because that's what symptoms are.

Furthermore, there is no way on earth to prove that a patient *avoided* ill health thanks to treatment. Try designing a research project on that and you'll come up with all sorts of problems. Those are issues for researchers to get to grips with.

So, it is true that we have a problem proving to the outside world that what we do 'works' except in a very shallow sense. And we also have a great deal of trouble from sceptics and other busybodies. One dear colleague was struck off because somebody somewhere didn't like the very reasonable information on his website. The Advertising Standards Authority decided they were unsubstantiated claims, and it seemed as if the regulator was then obliged to act.

Importantly, no patient had complained about his actual performance. He could have adjusted his wording but felt that the truth was worth defending. He received an outpouring of support from the profession and from patients, a firm signal of how at odds with good sense the regulatory process has become. I was dismayed that the regulator seemed to have no status as an authority except to punch down at an individual practitioner. We don't need that, and nor do the public. A number of us gave up our registrations after that.

But grown-ups don't need permission to spend their own money on something they feel instinctively to be good for them. And as long as we aren't reckless, dangerous, or deceitful, and the patient accepts the level of uncertainty involved, we have every right to deliver it.

The issue nobody is talking about is that if we focus on what works, by narrow, surrogate, outcome measures, then we might never know the true scope of our abilities. We could be making our patients sicker in the belief we were doing good. And my belief is that this is a problem across the entire healthcare spectrum. Just as worrying, some of the evidence we view as supportive might be invalid because it answers the wrong questions.

The flip side is that without nuance, we might show some highly effective treatments to be ineffective. It is hard to aim for excellence if all we have is a decidedly crude set of criteria for excellence—trial data, limited variables, higher or lower, true or false, best this, statistically that. We know it's a problem in education, but in healthcare it has got way out of hand.

Not only that, but we also risk being backed into corners by regulation or commercial dirty tricks.

So, what is the antidote?

Whether research findings appear to support our approach or not, we must distance ourselves from any research that cannot speak to our own aims in life.

What really matters is not how the patient is in thirty minutes. It's how they will be in a month, a year, ten years. Will they be able to play with their grandchildren? Will they be leading a productive life well into old age? It's nice to be told I am good at what I do, but I will only know for sure when I can start counting the patients who make it to 100.

If we don't want to wait that long, there are other ways we might approach the issue. The market speaks volumes, so we could begin by asking how many happy customers we have. People generally spend their own money on things that serve them in some way. Hospitals have many more customers than we do, but how many are so truly delighted with the service that they would be there without the state or an insurance company paying for it? I would bet a year's takings they are a very definite minority.

People go to natural therapists because they really do value the service. They feel the benefit, and they tell their friends, and their friends tell their friends. Then they get well, and we don't see them for years. And we frequently get things better for the price of a tank of petrol, that would have cost the taxpayer four or five figures taking the medical route. As a proportion of the millions we do see, those who feel it was worth it are, without a shadow of doubt, the majority.

"Oh, but they're self-selecting," say the critics, as if that means they aren't good witnesses.

Yes, self-selecting they are! Choice in therapy is important to good outcomes. Stop skewing the market and we'd see millions of others too.

"But people who go to natural therapists might be healthier to begin with. They don't need medical attention."

Do what healthy people do, and you might be healthier too.

"But we can't take their evidence into account, because they aren't reliable witnesses. They might just think they are better because of some placebo effect, or wishful thinking. It would skew our data."

In my view, nobody is more highly qualified to know if a therapy works than the patient. After all, they were qualified to know they were in trouble to begin with, and to seek professional help. The patient's subjective experience of suffering and relief is the doctor's reason for existing. If we can't take it into account, then what the heck is healthcare even for? But we do still have to look at broader outcome measures.

"But you're a practitioner. You have a subconscious bias. We can't take your word for it either."

If someone's scientific conclusions depend on practitioners deluding themselves, then they need to test that hypothesis. The research isn't complete until the mismatch between one set of perceptions and another has been investigated. Excluding our viewpoint is the real bias.

But I am also a patient. Moreover, I am an *expert* patient. And I do what I do because it's also what I want for me and my family. And I am personally very happy to be a patient of my own therapy. How many gastroenterologists, neurologists, dermatologists, oncologists, or colorectal surgeons would say that?

Researchers have, for whatever reason, been looking at this problem the wrong way around. Instead of observing the empirical truth that natural healers are hugely popular, and then analysing why that is, they have started by measuring the effectiveness of certain isolated techniques, applied in a prescriptive manner, and then come up with a theory of ineffectiveness. They have then had to deny the testimony of millions of good witnesses in order to support their position.

We need to be sure we don't fall for it, or worse, make the same mistake.

[1] Michael Nevradakis, PhD, *'Brought to You by Pfizer': Pharma Giant Spends More on Ads, News Sponsorships, Than Research*, The Defender, 2 Nov 2021, https://childrenshealthdefense.org/defender/pfizer-vaccination-ads-news-sponsorships-research/.

[2] Jennifer Jones, *10 Largest Lobbying Groups in the United States*, Largest, 4 Dec 2019, https://largest.org/people/lobbying-groups/.

[3] World Health Organisation, *Who funds the World Health Organisation?* https://www.weforum.org/agenda/2020/04/who-funds-world-health-organization-un-coronavirus-pandemic-covid-trump/.

[4] *U.S. Judge Finds Medical Group Conspired Against Chiropractors*, New York Times, 29 Aug 1987, https://www.nytimes.com/1987/08/29/us/us-judge-finds-medical-group-conspired-against-chiropractors.html.

[5] Joseph Mercola, *How fact checking is controlled and faked*, https://articles.mercola.com/sites/articles/archive/2022/02/09/fact-checking-controlled-and-faked.aspx.

[6] Sharyl Attkisson, *Astroturf and manipulation of media messages*, Ted Talk, https://youtu.be/-bYAQ-ZZtEU.

[7] Dr Malcolm Kendrick, book, *The Great Cholesterol Con*.

Missing Link 2: A coherent roadmap to recovery

This guy's doctor told him he had six months to live.
The guy said he couldn't pay his bill. The doctor
gave him another six months.

—Henny Youngman

It might seem self-evident that a healer's job is to heal the patient, but for a number of reasons, I would disagree with that.

For one thing, the highest goal is, in fact, to do no harm. If you can slow the progress of a problem or even reverse it, so much the better. Improving their situation is fairly far down the list and total resolution is sometimes not achievable. Alas, target fixation—aiming for measurable improvement above all else—can upset our priorities. But if you can make life a little better, in some way, for most of your patients, and don't do any harm, then you are already doing a great job.

For another, it is nature's job to heal the patient, not ours. We can't do it, doctors can't do it: only nature can do it. Our job is to clear the obstacles.

There is also a belief that doing good must have some kind of downside; that an effective treatment is one where the benefit outweighs the risk. "You can't make an omelette without breaking eggs," some would say. In fact, that need not be so. It is very possible to work in a way that is highly tolerant of error, by simply promoting health as the best solution to disease.

For example, if somebody needs a glass of water, there is no downside to giving them a glass of water. The issue is in determining what the person actually needs, not merely what will make them feel better in the moment. By addressing their true needs, their suffering is relieved as a matter of course, and there is no real downside.

Researchers in various fields, both sympathetic and hostile, have occasionally tried to quantify the dangers of spinal manipulation. I find nearly all the work in this area deeply unconvincing and often heavily biased. And indeed, it is possible to do anything in life dangerously, including manipulation … and including drinking water. Past efforts to find evidence of serious harm have required dredging the literature for anecdotal evidence, much of it from malpractice cases. Given the millions of people who go to osteopaths and chiropractors every week all over the world, the numbers for serious adverse events are reassuringly low, if anything.

Whilst it is certainly possible to make somebody worse through natural therapy, it is also possible to avoid doing so with the right training and experience. True harms are therefore avoidable, even if they aren't necessarily avoided; unlike with medical drugs, where harm is simply a numbers game, and a large attrition is inherently unavoidable.

More than 100,000 people are killed in the USA each year by medical drugs, just in hospitals [1]. Outside of the hospital, who knows? That's just the ones prescribed and used properly, and where the connection between the drug and the fatal complication has actually been recognised. I believe many more are overlooked, ignored, or positively swept under the carpet, and this number doesn't include accidental or intentional overdose or prescribing errors. And that's just the drugs. Medicine overall is now widely understood to be the third leading cause of death in the United States, after heart disease and cancer [2]. The patterns can't be so very different in other countries. Some deaths may defy categorisation; for example, death in recovery from an operation following a heart attack that might have been caused by painkillers. Most likely it would be recorded as a cardiovascular case. So, there may be no way to tell just how high the numbers are, but they are high.

The point is, millions of deaths over time are seen as the acceptable downside, a necessary price to pay for the practise of medicine. They have committees working it all out: how many will be saved versus how many will be killed, if they give a certain drug to a thousand cases, and whether it is worth it according to some value set. In that world, one might easily develop a sense that everything is a risk/benefit balance.

The number of natural healers I know personally who are even suspected of having had a dead patient on their hands is precisely zero. And in the profession worldwide, it is statistically so close to zero as to really bring into question whether risk of death is an issue in our business. It is possible that our treatment even extends lives; not something anybody has really looked into. But since our purpose is health, why not?

There are also people out there determined to show that spinal manipulation has no benefit. And in a sense, that is correct. Neither spinal manipulation nor any other isolated technique do anything in their own right, just as boxes of spanners don't fix cars without a mechanic to guide their use. A study on 'spannering cars' would only prove that spanners are useless. We should therefore be really careful when identifying therapies by their methods, since the method should not be the therapy.

But there are many therapies where the method is the defining feature: massage, herbalism, dry needling, chiropractic, for instance. I can think of only a few that are defined by their blueprint for human health. Osteopathy is supposed to be one of them. It's a shame that many practitioners reject the idea of a blueprint and lean almost entirely on a loosely specified collection of methods to define their work. Some even lean on the title alone, saying vapidly, "Osteopathy is what an osteopath does", meaning, as far as I can tell … anything goes. And thus, the mechanics spend their time discussing spanners rather than engineering, laying them open to accusations that they don't really have much of a plan to get people better. And the lack of a strategy is a problem, as I will explain shortly.

In fact, among all the professional skills and qualities listed by healthcare regulators as necessary—taking a case history, examining the patient, administering treatment, interpreting data and so on—nowhere does it mention actually getting people better. I wonder why.

But the point is that we should not be trying to balance risk against benefit at all. We should be looking for solutions that raise health and therefore have no downside. It need not even be difficult. It just means following a coherent roadmap that is broad and patient-centred, rather than a disease-centred, reactive, and direct approach that is based only on the name of the condition, or on the practitioner's favourite techniques. Patient-centred and indirect approaches don't rely on the same critical accuracy as when one commits to treating strained and inflamed structures directly with a predetermined technique. At the very least, this makes indirect approaches somewhat tolerant of error—more likely to do no harm.

Some therapists already have their idea of a roadmap. But for those who don't, I'm offering one here. The overall strategy behind it all is remarkably straightforward: remove stress from your patient and then wait. Respond to the events that then unfold, as if they are healing processes to be supported, not opposed. Repeat as required. Create healthy conditions and health will emerge if you let it.

The features of that roadmap—north pointer, signposts, forks in the road, landmarks etc—are in the other missing links. The healing crisis, terrain theory, the toxic state, and the progression and regression of disease, are particularly important for general navigation. They tell us which way to go when the destination is far over the horizon, and whether or not we are heading in the right

direction, even when the road is steep and winding. They
help us to avoid peat bogs and dead ends, or paths that
appear straight and smooth but eventually veer off in the
wrong direction. They help us know when to act, when to
wait, and when to send somebody off to the emergency
room.

So, we set off from the point where the patient asks
for help, and guide them towards a place called independence, teaching them the map as we go.

Exactly how we translate all that into tangible actions
is, of course, a lifelong study. But I will start here by urging you to feel your way into the problem, in stages if
necessary, and proceed with caution when encountering
any kind of resistance. If you don't get the change you
want, it means either the body isn't ready, or it's not the
change that's needed, so don't force it. Don't be tempted
by short cuts, and keep looking at the bigger picture
always. See how the body responds over time and then
adapt the approach accordingly. Hand over the reins to
the patient as progress allows.

Some days there will seem to be no progress, and every
journey has stretches like that. There are times when the
best decision is to do nothing and simply wait. That doesn't
mean there is no role for the practitioner. It means that the
practitioner needs a sense of strategy and timing.

It all works because the body has an intelligence and
always knows how to heal itself. The practitioner doesn't
have to cure anybody, just keep them on the right path.

In contrast, the roadmap handed down from medical philosophy is more like this. Diagnose the condition
or the symptomatic structure and infer your intervention

from that. When diagnosis fails, treat the signs and symptoms anyway, as they appear. Avoid any aspects that lack a clear relevance to the condition. Drive the disease out of the body and whatever remains will be health. Have a good legal plan.

It isn't hard to see why the medical roadmap is so riddled with problems. It isn't so much a roadmap as a repertoire of reactions to events encountered. It isn't surprising, therefore, that so many patients end up in quagmires or dead-ends, or sure-footedly going around in circles. And natural therapies are every bit as capable of taking a reactive approach.

Both patient and practitioner can choose which roadmap to follow. But I would argue that you can't follow both. You can't flit between them. On the choice of roadmap, there must be agreement between all parties, including other practitioners, or the relationships will not be therapeutic or lasting.

I would further argue that it is not possible to mix roadmaps between one holistic therapy and another. For one thing, that wouldn't be holistic, and there is far more to why that matters than just ideological purity. Healing can be a bit of a rollercoaster, as symptoms change or move around. New symptoms may appear, and old ones may return for a while. The body's healing reactions can themselves be startling, at times. And there is no shortage of practitioners around willing to take a snapshot and jump on those developments, without necessarily any sense of the overall flow. When the going gets tough, there is no sense of oversight anywhere and the patient quickly reaches out to medicine—or to the nearest mystic.

Therefore, great confusion can arise when multiple therapies are involved, and sometimes all it takes to turn around a difficult case is to stop the patient from going to every healer in town. That doesn't mean other professionals aren't ever needed. It just means that therapy can't be treated as a smorgasbord of modalities bolted together. At the very least, there must be some navigational harmony, and alas, that is rare. Some integrated clinics try to deal with this by having a coordinator who directs the patient to the right modalities. But that is not the same as everybody singing to the same tune. In fact, one solid holistic practitioner can be worth an entire health resort full of modalities.

There will, of course, occasionally be times when only specialist intervention or emergency medical care will do, and it would be reckless not to call upon it if needed— one basic competency of any practitioner is knowing when they are getting out of their depth. The issue is not always that the therapist lacks a rationale to help. The point is that time runs out on those cases.

The bottom line is that healing is automatic. That removes an awful lot of pressure in our business. Creating the circumstances for recovery is the real trick. Keep that in mind and you will acquire a system that is versatile, tolerant of error, and highly effective.

[1] Lazarou J, Pomeranz BH, Corey PN. *Incidence of adverse drug reactions in hospitalized patients: a meta-analysis of prospective studies.* JAMA. 1998 Apr 15, 279(15):1200-5. doi: 10.1001/jama.279.15.1200. PMID: 9555760.

[2] Makary M A, Daniel M. *Medical error—the third leading cause of death in the US*, BMJ 2016; 353 :i2139 doi:10.1136/bmj.i2139.

Missing Link 3:
Spontaneous recovery

*The art of medicine consists of amusing the patient while
nature cures the disease.*

—Voltaire

I once heard an old Indian doctor pronounce in front of a large audience: "If you want to be well, stop doing the thing that is making you sick."

At first, I thought I had wasted my time going there. If this was supposed to be some kind of profoundly deep healing wisdom, then the guy's a charlatan. Surely after fifty years of medicine he can do better than that?

My initial discomfort and confusion were because he was right. As a patient, it meant I couldn't expect a product or service to help me, and it challenged me with things I knew one day I would have to face. And that meant I would have to make a monumental effort, not just with small things like drinking coffee and staying up late, but to deal with some profoundly huge issues in the way my life was structured, with absolutely no idea how to even begin solving those issues. In fact, for somebody who had recently trained in the business of offering solutions, this felt like a slap in the face.

But after a while, the message became truly empowering. He was offering a valuable gift. He was giving back to his audience what had been taken away from them, namely control over their own destiny in health. My discomfort was really about the scale of the problem, but once I realised I could break it down, take it in steps, then it seemed something really worth considering. Okay, there may be ten things going on, and I only have easy control over three of them. So, I can start on those. And there may be aspects to the problem which I could change with a little effort or help, and a decent therapist could perhaps lighten the load there. Then there may be a few things that could be changed given the will to do so, which might just mean waiting for the right opportunity. That seemed a lot easier than forcing the issues. And finally, there are the things beyond all control. And whilst I can acknowledge them, and the limitations they impose, I need not pressure myself into changing what cannot be changed: the rest ought to be enough. Besides, once I start getting to grips with the other things, the unchangeable ones might seem more changeable.

It is interesting that modern medicine concentrates on the part of the problem that is hardest to change and ignores the rest. It sees the rest as irrelevant. It is much easier to sell a case for researching the genetics of incurability than to get to grips with the earthy nuts and bolts of the problem. Supposing I could close half the beds in a hospital with a few simple, tried, and tested things: who would pay me a million dollars to lead the way? And who in that hospital is going to be happy when it takes away their job? Will they even see any good in it?

The second big slap in the face came near the end of my training, when I met an American practitioner, who told a few of us over dinner: "You guys need to understand that you aren't going to heal anybody."

This was an even bigger challenge to the ego. Why would we be in this business if we weren't going to make people better? Speak for yourself, matey!

Again, after time, this dismal news turned into a profoundly empowering message. The point is not that we can't get people better, it's that we don't even need to. They get better by themselves. We don't have to cure them, Mother Nature does that, and she does a better job than any of us can dream of. Furthermore, she works in ways that humans can barely understand. And our role is to remove the obstacles to healing and create the conditions for recovery, then step out of the way and let nature do her work. The more we interfere, the less room there is for natural recovery.

Recovery is, in fact, the all-important word to hold on to. Not cure, not healing: those things are a myth, at least in the direct sense of the practitioner fixing the patient. There is nothing to fix. If the patient is alive, they are already perfect. Their system is doing the very best it can under the circumstances. It's the circumstances we need to fix, and if we can do that, then some degree of recovery is inevitable, providing they are not in their final hours.

Another key concept that we almost never discuss outside of academic situations is homoeostasis—the self-maintaining ability of all living things. Homoeostasis is one of those missing links that is hiding in plain

sight. There is a dynamic state of balance and equilibrium to life that I will go into later, which means that,
within certain limits, the human body will always right
itself, like a spinning top. If the top falls over before
it stops spinning, it is because it has hit a notch in the
table.

Another word we hear but seldom give much significance is thermodynamics. Living systems are arranged so
that they always seek the lowest energy state, at all times.
As much as they are arranged to produce energy and use
it in great bursts if needed for survival, or reproduction,
or to create a better life for themselves, the aim of doing
so is always to return to the state that uses the least energy
to maintain the living equilibrium, since that is the most
stable and enduring possible arrangement.

*In short, the human body seeks health as surely as water seeks
the lowest point, and it only stops when it hits an obstacle. So, our
job is to clear the obstacles.*

A body expressing symptoms of illness is already in,
or seeking out, its lowest energy state for whatever it
is dealing with. As soon as we try to 'cure' the system,
we are in fact taking it out of its arrangement of choice
and demanding the body do more work. Most direct
approaches to treatment do this. They achieve a localised
result but make more work for the system overall. When
vitality is low (a concept I will cover later), this can be
catastrophic.

In an extreme example, when a person is in intensive
care, there may be direct intervention in anything unusual
the body is trying to do. It is felt that the person is in
such grave danger that anything outside of normal could

kill them and must be corrected. So, they measure fifty different things and if something is high, they try and bring it down. If something is low, they bring it up. If something is irregular, they try and stabilise it. If there is a bacterium, they try to kill it. If they haven't had a bowel movement, they give them laxatives. The idea is that if all the measurements can be steered close to normal and held there for long enough, then the patient will be closer to recovery.

The issue here is that the demands this places on a body may cause further stress and complications, as it isn't ready for those things to be normal. If the patient still dies, then of course it was because they were so gravely ill, and "We did everything we could for them." Maybe *doing less* would have been better.

The more day-to-day example would be a fever, when it is wrongly believed, both by the public and by many medical practitioners, that fever is dangerous and must be brought under control with drugs (more on that later). But the fever is already under control, even high fever. It hasn't happened by accident: it is one of the tricks the body can use to solve a problem, and it knows what it's doing. The issue for the therapist is once again whether simply bringing the fever down will be helpful. Usually, it isn't.

What might be considered pathology is really *hyperphysiology*—the body doing extraordinary things under extraordinary circumstances. When the event is over, those way-out parameters will return to normal by themselves, if they need to.

Even medical doctors are now remembering this. Many developments in Intensive Care theory and practice in recent times have involved doing less for the patient, and they are saving more lives that way [1]. They have found that, even in extreme situations, the most important thing is still to provide a safe and supportive environment for the patient, and anything else is a bonus. As long as the airways are clear, blood is circulating, kidneys are filtering, ducts aren't blocked, the nervous system is alive, and there is no pressure on the organs, the best thing is often to let the body get on with sorting itself out.

So, it's no surprise that in the less glamorous world of natural healing, the more experienced we get, the more we seem to see patients getting better on their own. Sceptics sometimes latch onto this, saying most of our success is down to spontaneous recovery. Well, I hope all of it is. When new to the business, one often feels a failure if the patient isn't better straight away. But this isn't always realistic. The real sign of success is when they stop coming and you wonder why, and you bump into them a few months later and they say, "The problem went away on its own and I've been fine ever since." Those are outcomes I'm often proud of, but it can be a lonely victory.

The fact is, there is no other kind of recovery. We can offer benefit and support. A surgeon can reunite the sides of a wound. But the only real healing is spontaneous, arising out of the natural physiological processes of the living body. Once dead, you are dead, and nothing can turn that around. And so, for the medical or healing practitioner, creating the conditions for recovery, whether through brilliant surgical repair, or by removing stress imprints from the system somehow, or by promoting behavioural and environmental changes, or by neutralising some toxin, or offering some missing nutrients, is all we can really do. Occasionally, we have to manage some kind of process, but that usually means observing and waiting.

And it is all medicine can really do as well. Most doctors would agree that without the natural healing power of the body, their treatments are limited, at best. But saying it is one thing and staking one's outcomes on it is quite another. They then hit the body with drugs to control something directly. They expect a pill to fix the malfunctioning body, while the patient's circumstances go unchanged. If they give you more than one pill, they might even call it holistic.

Natural healers have to face a lot of scepticism. Many think we believe in magic and superstition. If anything is trying to operate outside of the laws of science and nature, it is the drug-based medical model. The laws of thermodynamics say, loosely, that you can't get something for nothing, yet that is exactly what modern medicine proposes. Take the pill and carry on. Your disease will just go, leaving only health behind. No need to change a thing. But we all know it can't possibly work that way. The very word 'pharmacy' derives from the Greek word for witchcraft.

The term 'natural therapy' should automatically imply respect for evolved biological constraints. Why anyone thinks this means magic is beyond me. But there is a fine line between asking enough of nature or too much, which drugs usually cross, and which natural therapists easily can cross when focused on conditions and isolated parameters. There are very few clues when observing a practitioner at work. You can watch a bridge being built and think you understand it because you see the bricks and mortar going together. But there are things going on in the minds of the architects and engineers that are not obvious even from their drawings. You can take those same bricks and put them together in a way that falls down.

This is why some practitioners can display impressive technical ability, and even bring great initial relief, yet still fail to deliver on that most important outcome—independence. Their patients may believe utterly in them and tell others all about the sense of benefit they get every single visit, but be no better a few months later, or even be worse. Others just seem to have an effortless ability to get people better. The difference is not technique, but vision.

During my first few years in practice, I would be deeply disappointed if the patient left the room without saying he felt amazing. Later on, I realised that the ones who didn't feel much different at first were often those who felt far better in a few sessions than they had for years. Importantly, they also didn't slip back.

Sometimes the most impressive results come from the most unimpressive treatment. Good healing should be boring and often is. The hallmark of mastery in any field is making something look easy, as if there is nothing to it. And after twenty years in practice, healing should be easy most of the time. If not, then the chances are that yet another course in advanced technique isn't the answer. What's needed is a different way to think.

If recovery is the concept we need to hold on to, then how do we consider the processes through which it works, so that we can be guided in cultivating the conditions for it, in recognising the conditions that work against it, and when necessary, to steer it? Read on.

[1] Dan Jones, *Darwinian medicine: Does intensive care kill or cure?* New Scientist 11 Aug 2010, https://www.newscientist.com/article/mg20727731-600-darwinian-medicine-does-intensive-care-kill-or-cure/.

Missing Link 4: Progression and regression of disease processes

For every complex human problem, there is a solution that is neat, simple, and wrong.

—H. L. Mencken

O ne of medicine's most profound secrets is hiding in plain sight. It resides in words used commonly in medical settings, whose meanings are in black and white in any medical dictionary, but the true importance of which is almost universally unrecognised.

An 'acute' condition is defined as one that comes on suddenly, often with severe, but short-lived symptoms, or one having severe symptoms and a short course. This is in contrast to 'chronic', from the Greek 'khronikos', meaning to do with time.

Chronic does not mean more severe (although it can signify deep-seated problems): it means persistent or long-standing. The line between acute and chronic is sometimes arbitrarily set at three months, or six, or some other number, and we were taught in college that chronic problems don't yield to treatment very easily. But beyond that—and the general understanding that chronic problems can be highly unrewarding to deal with—the monumental significance of these terms was barely addressed.

What is staring us in the face is that acute problems get better on their own. That is their very definition. I should say, they get better on their own, providing they don't kill you, and in practice, the vast majority don't. With a recent onset, very little treatment is needed, usually, except perhaps to help things along, and unnecessary treatment can in fact make matters much more complicated. As long as the event that caused it has passed and there is no ongoing threat or damage to the tissue structure, then there may be very little to do except wait.

If an acute episode is a repeat of something that has been re-occurring for many years, or the cause isn't clear, then there may be a less visible chronic situation behind it—an ongoing source or pattern of stress that imprints itself upon the body. In those cases, work is needed, but is often best left until the acute event is over. And I'll explain why shortly.

There is better news still, and this isn't stated in any modern medical textbook. And that is, after a well-managed acute episode, the patient can actually feel better than they did before. According to C Leslie Thompson: "This … is less credible to the orthodoxly thinking person who hears of friends 'weakened by a series of illnesses'. In the latter case, a truer description would be 'weakened by a series of suppressive treatments'." [1]

But so far, I am still just setting the stage. We were taught that an acute problem that doesn't go away becomes chronic, but the reasons given were vague. And because chronicity is harder to treat, many of my colleagues quite openly say that they prefer to treat only acute cases. It is generally accepted that chronic cases require management rather than treatment, since they are unlikely to be resolved at all and can only be relieved for a time. And I have seen many patients with chronic problems discharged by their practitioners for the sole reason that they had nothing to offer them that might make life a little better.

"Oh, but there's degeneration," they say. Well, of course: tissue change, and loss of tissue health, are hallmarks of chronicity. In effect, we have been saying collectively that we can only treat things that don't really need much, if any treatment at all, and we can't treat the things that do. And we will dump onto doctors those problems for which doctors don't have real solutions either, and call it *best practice*. Practitioners are even known to use terms like 'heart-sink patient' among themselves. It's a shameful state of affairs.

The next golden nugget is this. Acute problems *that are not properly managed*—that are suppressed, over treated, not supported, or cut short through lack of opportunity to play out—are the ones that become chronic.

And finally, most important of all for the therapist, is that *chronicity resolves through acute episodes.*

It is chronicity that is the real opportunity for treatment. It is chronicity that deserves the most attention: if we are going to push anywhere, chronicity is where we really need to push. If, in actively treating the chronic, we can enable an acute event to start by itself, then the chronic patient has a chance of lasting improvement.

Confused? I'll simplify that. *Acute needs good management, and chronic needs good treatment; the exact opposite of what many believe.*

Hence, back to the original example of shingles, this is why it may actually be best to do nothing but wait. Even if that means a spell of discomfort for the patient, the consequences of offering short-term relief will eventually be worse. But the silver lining is that the acute episode will be beneficial in the end.

And here is why. Acute effects are survival or healing processes, often the immediate reaction of the body to some kind of threat or insult, with the aim of rejecting or neutralising that problem and preventing it from causing real harm. Anybody who has ever had too much vodka knows that the acute reaction is to vomit. However unpleasant it may be, we all understand why it is necessary and why it shouldn't be stopped. It eliminates the toxins and prevents them from building up in the tissues, or worse.

The person who is so poisoned that they cannot vomit is in real danger. Yet it isn't unusual in care home and hospital settings to administer anti-emetic drugs when, for some strange reason, they can't keep down institutional food and medication, or the ghastly cocktails fed down a hair-fine tube through the nose which, alas for some, may be the only way to eat. In those situations, vomiting is seen as the problem, and not the nauseating substances being provided. The body's failure to tolerate the diet can apparently be fixed with a drug. If that style of management is kept up, of course the body will try to adapt, since it needs to mitigate the harm of these irritants as best it can. And in the process, the patient's vitality will be consumed at a high rate. In time, they will get sicker, and along will come the drug for that as well.

The right solution ought to be better diet and less medication, one might think. But try getting that across in an institutional setting. I have ...

The threat need not always be external, it can include prior internal build-up of waste or other unfinished business of repair.

Terms like *'sub-acute'* and *'acute-on-chronic'* refer to various states of grumbling chronicity. There may be too much going on for a completely cathartic acute storm to be raised safely, but the body still has the reserves of energy needed to try. Little attempts at acute activity will bubble up from time to time, usually to be driven back down again with some kind of suppressive drug or technique.

And so, almost any acute symptom you can think of is a protective mechanism or a healing process, and should not be regarded as a malfunction in any way. Runny noses, achy limbs, and fever, are all natural physiological effects. These common cold and flu symptoms are signs of healing attempts, not signs of failure to heal. Similarly, sore backs, sore throats, coughing up green goo, boils, diarrhoea, earwax, tears, rashes, anger and anxiety, hair loss, piles, cloudy urine, smelly poo, fatigue and lethargy, fear, punching a mugger on the nose ... all can be traced to the body's attempts to

survive as long as possible. Strong symptoms do not
have to mean a more severe problem: a strong body
can react strongly, but weakened bodies tend to react
weakly.

And inflammation—almighty inflammation—is how
we repair diseased and damaged tissue. It literally stops
us from falling apart. And yet suppressing inflammation
is a vast industry. The pain is there to warn you: Stop!
Something is wrong, and we are closed for repairs. But
inflammation provides other important services besides
warning you not to use the bit that's in trouble. If you
interfere with those repair processes—and worse, numb
the inflamed part and keep working it—you are on the
road to severe damage.

Still, the body won't give up, though. It will adapt as
best it can. It may come back with more inflammation,
more pain, leading to stronger drugs and so on. This
is one important way that a chronic problem becomes
established. Once the adaptations set in, you become
stuck with it more permanently. You won't necessarily
feel it at first. What you will feel is when every so often
the body tries again to resolve the issue, and to dump
the associated baggage it has acquired on the way. And
of course, if your habit and that of your doctors is to
suppress symptoms, then the chances are you won't know
any different. You will keep suppressing and keep digging the chronic hole, and all the while be grateful for the
diminishing effect of palliative measures.

If it seems that the point is to suffer the full brunt
of inflammation without any kind of mercy from the
therapist, it isn't. The aim of the holist isn't to make

inflammation go away, but to remove the reason it is needed in the first place. Meanwhile, the process can be made more comfortable by supporting it to a quick and complete resolution, as opposed to simply switching it off.

Adequate Vitamin D levels and good nutritional status—things a long hospital stay can challenge—are vital to stop inflammation getting out of hand. Large doses of Vitamin C given evenly over time are not only supportive but, in my view, necessary [2]. Resting affected tissues is imperative, since loss of function is characteristic of inflammation. And when used properly, careful bodywork, 'drawing out' compresses, and heat, can really help. Caution is needed with heat, however, since there are pitfalls and contraindications, and misuse can sometimes make matters worse. Ice packs are usually a waste of time, and you won't find one in my office.

Not only have I seen this approach bring great relief, it has worked in situations when suppression has already failed. The same approaches that help ease and resolve inflammation can do the same for some cases of infection (or 'outfection', as it should be called—discussed later). But I would stress that these are not times to go reinventing the wheel. If doctors are involved in the case, it is imperative to communicate your ideas with them, even if the response is sneering. My premise is that what we would have to do on a desert island, if it is safe, is usually going to help.

Some popular 'natural' adjuncts such as turmeric, may be essentially suppressive. It can be hard to tell. The idea of anti-inflammatory foods seems to fit the combative mindset of countering healing instead of supporting it. Avoiding pro-inflammatory foods, while providing antioxidant support, is a more appropriate way to view this. The current popularity of so-called adaptogens—supplements that promote adaptation—seems to be completely missing the point, which is to remove the causes of disease, rather than develop a tolerance.

Of course, an inflamed organ is a serious matter. But merely suppressing the inflammation is not a long-term solution. Acute pancreatitis (inflamed pancreas), they say, leads to chronic pancreatitis and then pancreatic cancer. Well, does it? Or is it the medical treatment that causes the progression? And what of the original cause? I don't advocate ignoring an inflamed pancreas: my point is we need a much smarter way to get to grips with the problem, and this is definitely an occasion when there needs to be a decent doctor onboard. I would not mention pancreatitis had I not actually known somebody who resolved their own chronic pancreatitis without drugs and was still fine many years later. I am not here to tell you how, just to say that dangerous chronic illness does not have to mean incurability and a lifetime of drug management.

Chronic disease may be invisible until fairly advanced. What we usually see are the acute attempts at resolution. Clues to chronicity's presence may be found sometimes in medical tests, but not always. Chronicity may leave us generally below par, and without always a clear description of the problem. But it creeps in, and as we adjust our habits around it, it can be passed off as our normal, or the effect of ageing. It can be our body's attempts to reverse it that we feel most strongly as a definite symptom picture.

Almost all effective medical treatments are for symptom management, and many of those work by suppressive means, driving the problem deeper in but without addressing cause. And this is one way—a major way—to make acute fail. And when chronic tries to resolve itself through further acute, it gets hit with further suppression. Quite simply, this is the medical approach.

But we can also acquire habits that suppress. Overwork, caffeine, strenuous exercise, various kinds of recreational stimulation, can all drive the fight or flight systems of the body. Conflict-seeking behaviour can do it as well, in, say, an angry or overly argumentative personality. And, as I will explain in a later chapter, these can all have a powerful suppressive effect, at least until the patient has completely exhausted himself. Once exhaustion is reached, the crash can be hard to bear.

Persistence of cause will also prevent resolution and lead to chronicity. And so, an important focus in therapy is to address the main drivers of the problem, which is often a case of fixing the roof when the sun is shining. But it is difficult to sell. "Come back when you're feeling better, and I'll treat you," can sound like ineptitude. But the cause of our back pain is not the bulging disc or stuck facet joint. The cause of the back pain is the complex set of circumstances that mean stress is focused on the disc or facet. And the most challenging time to overcome that can be when things are seriously inflamed.

So, the first point of management is to get the patient to obey their symptoms, even if that means they do nothing for a month. The alternative might be two months recovering from surgery.

The cause of asthma is not a constricted airway: it is the normal physiology of the body being over-amplified for some reason. The middle of an asthma attack is a bad time to sort out the causes, and if an inhaler is the only tool available, then it is silly not to use it. That said, dehydration can be a major exacerbation for asthma, and I have seen an attack stopped with a pint of water. It is certainly hard to say that suffocation is good for survival. But the process of asthma does, nevertheless, arise out of natural survival mechanisms, and at some point, we need to talk about how things get that far. Suffice to say, prior suppression or tampering with the natural immune system are normally in the history.

The challenge for the practitioner is to know whether a sudden eruption of symptoms signifies a change for the worse or for the better, or whether it needs watchful waiting or urgent action. Genuinely new problems can indeed arise during a course of treatment. Recently, I was treating a young man for a shoulder injury, when out of nowhere he developed appendicitis and was admitted to hospital. Something didn't seem quite right, and so the family called me. It didn't take long to realise this was not a normal post-treatment soreness. Interestingly, since I had last seen him, he had fallen off his motorbike, and the abdominal pain started some weeks later. After he got out of hospital and the surgery had healed, they brought him to me to continue treatment where we had left off. I found something new—his pelvis was jammed into a slight twist, presumably by the accident. The joints on the right of his pelvis and low back were rigid, meaning his entire low back and abdomen were not moving quite as they should.

Could that have affected the health of the appendix? Conceptually, yes it could, but not provably. Could he have kept his appendix by much earlier correction? We will never know, and on a desert island I might consider it, but otherwise I wouldn't let such thoughts delay getting to the hospital. The point is to dispel fluffy notions that all acute problems will resolve by themselves in the end, and about recognising when things are not business as usual.

We have the homoeopaths and natural hygienists to thank for much of our understanding in this area. They observed the way disease states change over very long timeframes, even over generations. They understood that a series of apparently unrelated health problems can, in fact, be a natural progression, good or bad, of the same circumstance. And they gave us some tools to help work it out. Modern doctors seldom see illness and disease play out un-tampered with, since their job is to intervene.

Out of this understanding arose Hering's Law, after a homoeopath called Constantine Hering. Loosely speaking, it posits that when a chronic disease state becomes more serious, the manifestations will tend to move further up the body, or deeper in, or will affect more important structures and functions. As things improve, the pattern reverses: the focus will tend to move down the body, outwards, affecting less important structures and functions. This recovery may take place in steps; either following treatment, or as a series of healing crises (explained later), or both. Importantly, the different stages may appear completely unrelated to each other, or as entirely separate conditions.

Straight away, this gives us a handle on where we are in the healing process, and whether or not our therapy is truly helping resolution or merely displacing the effects. It can give confidence, when the patient's complaints seem never-ending, that things are still moving in a positive direction, and it can also tell us when an urgent change of tack is needed.

An accessible example might be the person who sprains an ankle and seems to recover from it. But the slight alterations to the posture and gait throw a stress pattern into the spine that goes all the way to the top. The first we may hear about it is when they come to us for neck-related headaches.

As things worsen, once the physical realm has been swamped, the manifestations will become mental, and then finally emotional. And on the return journey, emotional symptoms will become mental, mental will become physical, and so on.

One last, very important feature of Hering's Law is that problems resolve in reverse order to how they came: old symptoms can return as more recent ones begin to ease. We can easily fail to register these progressions, seeing isolated aspects of the case out of context instead.

So, it is not uncommon for a patient with, say, headaches or sleep problems, to experience the return of an old neck, shoulder, throat, or chest symptom. Or they may get a head cold as something is eliminated through the sinuses. They may have forgotten all about the ankle they once injured, but now they find it sore to walk on. The trick is to then treat the lower problems without driving it all northwards again.

Not mentioned by Hering, as far as I know, but something I have observed, is that during recovery, a patient's problem will also often seem to simplify. It will become more localised, perhaps even more intense for a while. This is where some clinical training is important for evaluating the situation. It may take on a more definite form. The drivers will become more readily identifiable.

Understanding these progressions gives us a powerful handle on where we are in the journey, and which direction things are heading. From that, we can infer whether to treat or to manage.

When a patient starts complaining of new problems, it is very tempting to get drawn right into the minutiae and lose all perspective. It is a good idea to zoom out and go back over the entire history and see what patterns emerge. When something doesn't seem to fit, then you have a better idea of where to go with it. A good question to ask is: "Has this ever happened before?" Another is: "Would you be willing to swap this new problem for the old one?" If they would rather go back to how things were a month earlier, then something might be wrong. The chances are they will say, "Heck no, that was worse: I'd rather keep this." If the patterns of their chronic state really are unravelling as they should, they won't have to keep it for very long.

[1] C. Leslie Thomson, pamphlet, *The Healing Crisis*.
[2] Andrew Saul PhD, book, *Doctor Yourself*.

Missing Link 5:
The toxic state (and why we need to talk about viruses)

A new scientific truth is usually not propagated in such a way that opponents become convinced and discard their previous views. No, the adversaries eventually die off, and the upcoming generation is familiarised anew with the truth.

—Max Planck

My postgraduate teacher told me, "Your first duty as an osteopath is to address the toxic state." This startling statement wouldn't compute for most osteopaths trained to think of theirs as a musculoskeletal discipline. Toxicology got very little space in our curriculum. If we suspected poisoning, we would have referred a patient to a doctor, but obvious and severe examples would generally not come to us, anyway.

Milder, every day toxicity wasn't discussed much either, and therapeutic 'detoxing' wasn't really seen as very relevant to our discipline. I've always been aware of it: but my first duty? That was news to me as well.

In any case, most people seem fairly aware of the importance of limiting exposure to artificial chemicals. But in fairness, most will try to find some kind of compromise; after all, we must keep our homes and gardens neat, and most of all avoid germs, because they're the worst, right?

For some, the balance means not having in their house anything that might accumulate in their tissues. For others, it means not getting too much glyphosate on their feet while weeding the lawn. Restaurants have, in recent years, toned down the 'squirt and smear' style of cleaning that placed speed above real hygiene. That's more likely because diners didn't appreciate being enveloped in a cloud of disinfectant, than because of any understanding that a wet cloth is actually better.

Agricultural chemicals are something most people trust to be safe enough in the small amounts they hope are used, and either see them as a price to pay for affordable produce or don't think about them much at all. Food additives abound, we know, and we like to think we avoid them when we can; but the attitude is often that they haven't killed us so far.

Actually, I have literally met a cancer patient walking into Starbucks to celebrate her last round of chemotherapy, and another one leaning over a pub wall at midday with a big glass of wine and a plate of deep-fried dim sums, lamenting the return of his tumours. We all like to think we are onto it, but many of us really aren't.

The so-called 'Hygiene Hypothesis' has been used to explain the explosion of allergies in children. I don't buy it. The idea goes that when we avoid germs, our immune systems lack the training they need to be strong. This notion started during polio outbreaks, to explain why it was middle-class children who got polio … as if middle-class children never went into the garden and always washed their hands!

A far more likely cause of these more long-term deleterious problems is the antiseptic measures themselves. I see a kitchen counter covered in disinfectant as no safer than one covered in bacteria—less safe, in fact, since we have no mechanism for dealing with many petrochemicals.

And I have seen people carry on around a broken fluorescent tube without batting an eyelid, when the recommendation is to evacuate the area and call in a specialist. I have seen hospital cleaners bleaching and dusting all around a patient with severe lung disease. And this is just the tip of the iceberg. Thousands of residents in Auckland, New Zealand, complained of serious health effects after the entire city was sprayed for painted apple moth in 2002. One only has to walk around a supermarket to realise we are all being poisoned.

There remains a tension between us wanting to protect ourselves, and manufacturers of everything from toothpaste to modems trying to convince us that their new toxins are not as dangerous as the old ones, while more and more new household products pour onto the market every year. The days of heavy indoor smoking, leaded petrol, and DDT in the drinking water have passed, but the days of hormone-disrupting plastic softeners, aggressive oven cleaner that tears through lipids, antibiotics in the milk, and fire-retardants in the mattress are here. And the explosion in medication and vaccines ought barely to need a mention. As for the vaccines, suffice to say any-thing that is *designed to* provoke the immune system into a reaction would be the absolute prime suspect when something unexpected happens to the immune system, one would think.

In many ways, toxins are not really a missing link at all. We all know to avoid them if we can, even if most people have little idea what that really means.

But there are aspects to toxicity that are very misunderstood, and that really is a missing link. Mild or even severe cases of insidious toxic accumulation are usually medicalised as if they were some other condition and treated with drugs. In much the same way, nutritional deficiencies are often mis-attributed and treated with drugs.

Accumulation of toxins is a stress that results from almost every other kind of stress. There can be lactic acid in the muscles from the gym, or the inflammatory waste products from an injury, or a build-up of harmful metab-olites when certain nutrients in the diet are insufficient, or the suspended general cleaning that takes place when sleep-deprived, or whenever levels of the stress hormone cortisol are for any number of reasons kept unsustain-ably high. And these accumulations are a big part of the reason for many symptoms. We can breathe mountain air, own an organic juice bar, and do yoga in a summer meadow all day long, and still be making toxins.

"What are these mysterious toxins?" ask the critics. The vast majority are the waste products of our own metabolism. This is self-evident, since we have large organs to deal with them. And the question is, where do they go?

When things are on an even keel, we are well-rested, free of worry, properly nourished, hydrated, and with bowel and kidney working well, they leave the body, since those are the conditions in which our systems are tuned towards maintenance processes like absorption, assimilation, growth, repair and elimination.

As we get busy and our stress levels rise for one reason or another, our fight-or-flight systems are activated, and those tasks are put off, to a greater or lesser degree. At the same time, heightened muscular and cellular activity causes more waste to be produced, and so any excess backs up, and must be stored for dealing with later on. The consequence is that waste gets driven out of blood and into tissues, and from there it is packed into cells to ensure we aren't overwhelmed by our own waste products while coping with stress. At that level, the effect is usually mild or temporary, and is easily reversed. But if stress is sustained, the build-up can go on unseen for years.

Waste also gets pushed into the extremities to protect the organs. Water may follow to dilute it. This may be the beginnings of achy or itchy limbs, sore joints, weight gain and swollen extremities. We might become prone to infections and infestations. Wounds might be slow to heal, and ulcers may form. There may be effects on temperament.

From there, it can be packed down further, being pushed into joints and fatty tissues. Hence, arthritis of various kinds can begin in fingers and toes but progress to affect more proximal structures as that mechanism fills up. Medication to disperse these effects can lead to more widespread or central disease—the very thing those mechanisms are there to prevent. Eventually, new tissue must be formed to accommodate the waste and keep it well contained or even walled off. And thus begins the formation of various lumps and bumps, tumours, and eventually malignancies. Needless to say, there is every variation and things don't always go in the same order, but the principle of storage is what needs to be recognised.

It's a fundamental concept that our bodies cannot do more than one thing to 100% at the same time. When our organs are flat out processing what is incoming, they are too busy to eliminate waste. And when we are busy nourishing ourselves or getting rid of waste is not a good time to be working hard. Hence, the man who wakes up with an alarm clock, throws down breakfast before his digestion is ready in order to make time for a stressful commute, works hard to make a living, eats lunch at his desk, keeps going with coffee, then visits the gym on the way home, stays up late with a glass of wine or two catching up in front of some kind of screen, and finally 'relaxing' on the weekend with a hectic social itinerary, is toxic. It may not appear so at first. "He is so energetic and lives life to the full," people say. Importantly, he may think because he has managed it for so many years, that when the signs and symptoms appear of some problem, his lifestyle can't be the cause. He is unaware of the fuzzy thresholds of accumulation.

When the process is reversed, such as in a change of routine or location, or cleaning up a lifestyle, this can be when the accumulation really shows, as the body starts unpacking the toxins and removing them via the bloodstream.

In extreme cases, such as a cancer patient going on an aggressive detox, the effect can fatally overwhelm the body. Specialised therapies such as Gerson, have to employ methods to prevent that, which is why people with very severe disease should be extremely cautious and seek expert help when trying to fix such problems. For most of us who have not reached that stage, we will experience some kind of healing crisis and take it in our stride. The term 'Healing Crisis' is something I will discuss later; it refers to a spontaneous healing event that is often mistaken for a dangerous illness. It is only when the effects of this natural detoxification are misunderstood and mismanaged that we are in any real danger.

When the symptoms of waste accumulation or its reversal are treated as a condition in themselves, that is when the chronic state can actually be accelerated. The danger area here is using anything that will take the symptoms head on, that is, by suppressing these processes: which is why I never use even 'mild', over-the-counter medications. People often tell me they don't like to use them either, and will only do so 'when they have to', by which they mean when things are unbearable.

It is when things are most unbearable that self-medication is most dangerous. When things are so unpleasant that they think they literally can't survive without some kind of drug, is precisely when they need immediate professional advice before taking anything.

Most people, I would think, can tolerate a great deal of suffering if they know it is temporary, to a good end, and that they aren't in any real danger. Assessing this can be where the experience of the practitioner is invaluable.

That said, there are often plenty of ways to get more comfortable without drugs and without resorting to suppression of symptoms.

Where the virus fits in

Whenever a patient tells me they have had a virus, I try and find almost any other explanation besides a virus. Whatever they may think they have had, and even with a test result to confirm it, there are a number of very important reasons why a virus is the least probable explanation.

For one thing, tests for viruses are imperfect, and can be fooled, making the issues of false positives more than just a rare concern. You can test positive or negative, with or without symptoms. Having a cold or being pregnant, for example, could be enough to fool the test. The information supplied with viral tests says that 'other viruses' can produce false positives, which is another way of saying the test isn't really specific at all.

In the case of HIV (Human Immunodeficiency Virus, officially the cause of AIDS, i.e., Acquired Immunodeficiency Syndrome), a positive result is supposed to be confirmed by a second test. But is the second test any better?

Importantly, these tests do not pick up diseases directly, but chemical markers that supposedly indicate viral agents. They are surrogate measures, in other words, and say nothing about one's health. It is starting to look as if the very meaning of viral tests is based on a highly circular logic: we know the tests work because we have all these viruses, and we know we have all these viruses, because we have all these tests.

We do also have all these sick people, but in the case of AIDS, many of them were put on pre-emptive treatments and got sick later. And the side effects are very similar to the illness they are supposed to treat, so what is actually making these patients sick?

Some were sick before they got tested, but from what, really?

In New York in the 1980s, it typically followed months of partying with drugs such as amyl nitrate, which is notoriously damaging to the immune system.

In Africa, the context might be malnutrition and poverty, and any number of health problems there were getting picked up by the AIDS dragnet.

This was the background against which AIDS was first investigated, and it was originally considered a toxic problem, not a microbial one. Then medical politics got involved, as it often does.

As an entry point to the subject of HIV/AIDS and the problems with the very construct, see Brent Leung's documentary, House of Numbers [1]. You'll likely end up wondering what AIDS is really supposed to be. But it doesn't cover the real monster lurking within statistics, which once seen cannot be unseen. I'll explain it as simply as I can.

A test with 95% reliability will throw up 50,000 false positives for every million people tested (5%). If none of those people have the virus, then you have the impression of a huge outbreak where there is none. Even if one person in a thousand had the virus, they would still be outnumbered by the false positives, fifty to one. And if all those 'cases' have to be contact traced, and all the contacts tested as well, then suddenly you have an explosion of overdiagnosis and misdiagnosis. Does that seem familiar?

Even if the virus itself didn't exist, one could show a huge outbreak, simply by bringing a 'test' for it onto the market. Worse still, suppose the test is the only way to know the virus exists … Can you see where this is heading?

You can play with the numbers all you want, and the problem doesn't go away. This applies to all kinds of medical test—one reason I am generally against routine screening [2]—and presumably to drug testing in sport and forensic science of all kinds. At the very least, one should always have a clinical reason for getting tested, in my view. Since public health officials should know this, it begs the question why they are so keen to push mass testing for viruses. And why do doctors go along with it? Answering these questions is not my purpose, but the ramifications are huge.

In the case of influenza, somehow it has been decided that flu symptoms, with a negative test, don't mean flu, so it's called *flu-like illness*. On what basis? Furthermore, if someone with no symptoms can still have a positive test, what does that say for the causes of flu? Who can see the correlation between the symptoms and the test result? I can't. The most logical position is that flu isn't caused by a virus.

For some reason, people find this very hard to take in, but it is staring us in the face. It appears virologists have been so fixated on their own paradigm that they have never stopped to wonder if they should go right back to the drawing board. Their rationale is like saying red shirts cause a football team to lose, except if they wear blue shirts, or don't lose. But whichever way it is, shirts *must* have something to do with it. As a result, we see endless morphing of a bad theory to fit the facts as they appear.

In short, a logical person might wonder how on earth we ever came to thinking disease was caused by viruses. I wouldn't labour the point, except to show unequivocally that viruses are one link humanity wouldn't miss.

But it gets deeper. There is very little evidence that colds and flu are even contagious, any more than leaves falling off trees in autumn. Consistently, it has proved difficult or impossible to pass on a supposed viral illness under experimental conditions.

The most famous example is the Spanish Flu experiment of 1919 that took place in Deer Island Military prison near Boston [3]. Various versions of the story exist, but the essential points are the same. Sixty-two prisoners (some sources give a different number) were offered full pardons in exchange for being exposed to the 'deadly' illness. For weeks they were locked in the prison infirmary, and every effort was made to induce Spanish Flu. The final stage was having sick patients—already diagnosed with the illness—cough five times into their open mouths.

Have you guessed how many of these volunteers fell sick as a result?

Zero is the answer.

Not one got so much as a sniffle. The explanation was, of course, that these volunteers already had an immunity, having survived an earlier outbreak in the prison.

Exactly how nature endowed them with the strength to get through the earlier crisis without symptoms—so as to have been eligible participants—isn't fully explained. The possibility that contagion is a flawed theory doesn't seem to be on the medical radar at all. One person involved did get sick, however, and actually died—the doctor in charge of the infirmary.

Prolific astrophysicists Fred Hoyle and Chandra Wickramasinghe modelled the spread of influenza mathematically, then compared the predictions with real life [4]. The data on actual spread did not support the contagion model. The main correlates for influenza were geography and meteorology—where you are and what the weather is doing. Proximity to large groups of people seems to have nothing to do with it. Whether this evidence supports their main thesis—that flu viruses come from outer space—I am not sure. But it clearly doesn't support the belief that they come from our neighbours.

Illnesses obviously do happen in waves and clusters, which does need explaining. But there are so many obvious environmental associations that blaming it on some tiny invisible malevolence jumping from person to person seems to be clutching at the smallest of straws. So, even when several children get ill after a birthday party, I don't assume something is just simply 'going around'. I want to know about the location, the food they ate, the games they played, what the weather was doing, what other common factors there may be, besides their sheer proximity to each other.

There are various other theories as to why we get colds and flu. But they all essentially amount to an occasional burst of immune activity to clear waste from the body, whether this is spontaneous and seasonal, like trees losing their leaves, or whether in response to some kind of stress or insult. When damaged cells need to be replaced, they break apart, or are broken apart, and the debris transported elsewhere for removal or recycling. One retired doctor pointed out, the DNA-containing nuclei need special care, since chopped-up fragments of genetic material let loose around the body could cause havoc. So, the remains of the nucleus are wrapped up in pieces of the old cell-membrane to render them harmless. He believed these little DNA-containing packets, thought to be emerging from diseased cells, are what we call viruses, and their function has been wrongly identified as harmful.

Radiation has often been blamed for the damage. But flu has been documented for thousands of years. So, it might be radiation, but it isn't just radiation. It may be different things at different times, making a single cause hard to pin down. But all versions amount to cells dying, for whatever reason, and needing to be gotten rid of. That much at least seems consistent, virus or not.

Another hypothesis is that they contain chemicals of communication to warn other individuals of a threat, in which case they are called exosomes, and may be responsible for what we see as contagion. It is perfectly possible that they are, in fact, neither of those things, or that they aren't even abnormal. But the question of contagion remains, and of whether it is real or illusory. I get whole days where it seems everybody has right-sided neck pain. Is neck pain a virus? I don't think so.

It's very hard to know what those blobs really are, seen only in black and white in a dead and preserved sample inside an electron microscope. One thing they aren't, is exclusive to sick people. They are found in everyone, everywhere.

The fact is, we all have old cells that need removing from the body, and periodical bursts of this activity are as natural and normal as the seasons. So, we don't necessarily even need a theory of flu at all, any more than we need a theory of burping. We just need to obey what our bodies tell us at those times, and we'll be as fine as we can be.

Politically, socially, and economically, there is a great deal riding on the virus. That much should be obvious by now. But the history of virology itself is a tale of fierce competition between virologists and toxicologists.

Since before AIDS, polio outbreaks and even smallpox, there have been very soundly reasoned toxicity theories for viral illness. It just happens that they don't sell much in the way of chemical products. In fact, they tend to implicate chemical products. They lead to things that seem boring and expensive, like plumbing and water systems, and spoilsport measures like closing factories.

For instance, long before the herpes viruses were named, shingles was thought to be due to, among other things, arsenic, the origins of which were industrial, or medical, or in arsenate pesticides. This seems like a very reasonable explanation. Extending that idea, the toxins can enter the nervous system, from where it is not easy to get them out. The blisters and nerve pain appear when axoplasmic flow—chemical transport along the inside of a nerve cell—helps carry the toxins outwards towards the skin for elimination, thus clearing the brain and spinal cord. However unpleasant shingles may be, it's entirely possible this is how the body avoids encephalitis (brain inflammation). When encephalitis shows up in a shingles patient, it's perhaps because the shingles weren't enough, and not because the shingles caused it. Perhaps it is due sometimes to suppressive treatment internalising the toxins?

Epstein-Barr virus, blamed for glandular fever, also known as 'mono' (mononucleosis), is thought to precede Chronic Fatigue Syndrome (CFS). I have asked many patients with a CFS situation how their initial viral illnesses were treated, and always there has been the use of drugs to lower the fever, or antivirals, or both. So, we can't blame the virus alone. Furthermore, when I ask them about their history before the viral illness, the majority have had antibiotics at some point for an upper respiratory tract infection or an ear, nose and throat problem. I fail to see a virus here at all. Nor do I see a special syndrome. What I see is a predictable upwards progression to more difficult problems through toxic suppressive treatment, something I covered earlier. A toxic problem is how I see this, and when viewed in that light, some meaningful rationale for help can emerge.

This is a perfect example of why we can't we just think of our treatment in terms of benefits, risks and side-effects. We need to think in terms of how treatment influences the natural course of detoxification.

Polio paralysis was once thought also to be caused by heavy metals, in the spinal cord. That said, any number of toxins could be to blame for polio paralysis, such as the pesticide DDT, which was used by the truckload globally during the main polio years.

Measles and chickenpox seem, circumstantially, to be communicable, but that's a far cry from saying the mechanism is viral contagion. Despite what the press like to tell us, they are both pretty harmless. It was improvements in living conditions that saw the big reductions in measles death in the developed world, years before a vaccine was widely available. According to the World Health Organisation (WHO), "The overwhelming majority of measles deaths occur in countries with low per capita incomes or weak health infrastructures" [5]. The measles section of the USA's Centres for Disease Control (CDC) website notably omits this important point. Among the data the CDC present on domestic cases, hospitalisations and so on, measles death isn't mentioned [6]. I wonder why. Both WHO and CDC repeatedly emphasise the vaccine. They connect death with lower vaccination rates, an association that simply isn't supported by the facts [7], nor by the WHO's own mention of the clear association with poverty, nor by the near total absence of measles deaths in the USA, even in the unvaccinated.

A further problem is that guidelines in the UK use measles vaccination status as a factor in diagnosis [8]. In other words, if your child has been vaccinated, he is less likely to be given a measles diagnosis and recorded as a case, regardless of his symptoms. The obvious knock-on effect is that the role of the vaccine is exaggerated. This is embedded scientific error or even fraud, in my view.

The diagnostic guidelines in the USA no longer contain this error. But the fact that this obvious source of bias has been allowed to pass without challenge in Britain's National Health Service suggests that it may well be entrenched in medical perceptions generally; that if the child is vaccinated, look for another diagnosis first.

I have no desire to make a point about the vaccine, except that one cannot help noticing its indelible mark on everything. The point is that the subject of measles has itself become muddled.

If anybody reading this has the definitive proof that a virus really does cause measles, they stand to gain a large cash prize. Digging out the paper should take a doctor or scientist a few minutes at most—I mean, it's a medical fundamental, right? It could be the easiest 100,000 Euros you ever make. Contact a gentleman called Stefan Lanka for details. A medical student did once claim the prize and sued Dr Lanka when he refused to pay. The claimant won his case at first, but an appeals court overturned the decision.

Significantly, the court made clear they could not rule on the scientific arguments, and ruled instead on whether Dr Lanka could apply his own standards of proof. Those standards are available online, in German, for anyone to read and evaluate.

It is disappointing that the press has concentrated on the legal arguments and given practically no attention to the scientific ones. The question of whether viruses really exist is of massive public consequence: legal soap operas are not.

The big trouble with this entire subject is that it is impossible to evaluate from the outside. The only way to get far enough into it is to spend as many hours studying the same subjects as the experts; in the same institutions, sitting the same exams. Students who can understand it enough to critique it, and yet retain true mental autonomy, must be exceptions.

Such concentrations of authority do not serve mankind well. That is why it is vital that we each remain free to make our own determinations. Some of us will be wrong, and survival will be the judge.

The problem for the layman is where, even, to begin. Even experts in similar fields can have difficulty relating to each other's work. But the risks of us all thinking the same way are too great. Survival and advancement of a species depends on variation. If we must all think and act the same way in the face of every problem, then we are setting ourselves up for extinction.

At this time, I lean towards those who say it is up to virologists to demonstrate pathological viruses first, and the job of others to disprove second. The supportive science has been critiqued from various angles, and some of what is reported about the shoddy standard of work is frankly jaw-dropping [9] [10]. By definition, theories only exist when competition is permitted, otherwise they are dogmas. By that standard alone, virology appears closer to dogma.

Other explanations for common childhood illnesses have long been available. There is good reason to think they are in fact necessary developmental processes, perhaps signifying the switch of the infant immune system into the adult immune system. So why do we want to defeat them anyway, except out of fear? Many parents notice that children have growth spurts or other developmental leaps after these illnesses. And once they have happened, they don't need to happen again.

Curiously, you cannot get chicken pox and measles at the same time. You would think that if the body's 'struggle' against one could so reliably guarantee such absolute protection from the other, the body could stop either illness if it wanted to.

Zika virus was in the news a few years back. Various claims circulated on social media about the use of pesticides to control malaria in that region of South America. It appears they were even added to drinking water storage to prevent mosquito larvae from living there. If that was the true explanation for the explosion in horrifying birth defects, it may also explain why the expected spread throughout the Americas didn't occur.

There is a disease I had never heard of until I visited Australia, called Ross River Virus or Fever, which people say they have caught on camping trips in mosquito-infested areas. It has a variety of symptoms, which include muscle and joint pain or stiffness, rashes, swelling, fever, headaches, neurological problems, and fatigue. To prevent it, one is supposed to use insect repellent, such as DEET, exposure to which can sometimes cause musculoskeletal pain, rashes, swelling, headaches, neurological problems, and fatigue. Spraying of mosquito-prone areas with insecticide is not unusual either.

I am not in a position to say what definitely causes Ross River Fever or any other viral illness, but I am saying we should not fear competing hypotheses, and true scientists should welcome them. What I wonder is how the association with mosquito bites was noticed, since anybody visiting those parts of Australia is unavoidably bitten by mosquitoes ... I sincerely doubt there is any correlation.

We could apply this discussion, of virus versus toxin, to any viral illness known. But I have noticed a tendency for doctors to look to naturally occurring causes before man-made ones. And we as patients have been trained, since birth, to accept these explanations.

The thing is, toxicological solutions have a very poor return on investment, whereas virological ones concentrate countless billions into the pharmaceutical family. Viruses are also politically far more convenient than toxins. Governments can use such enemies to lever support for policy, and they like to hide bad news behind a crisis. Hence, virologists have always enjoyed better support, and in the war for hearts and minds, they have had the upper hand until now. They propose products that are easy to package and don't upset industry. The big question is whether they work. But since 2020, when governments went far beyond what was helpful, there is an increasing sense that public health has backed the wrong horse.

A logical way to confirm that a virus is the cause of a disease would start by showing it to be present in every clinical case, without cheating by re-naming the illness when the tests show negative.

Then one would have to show that the virus isn't present in any healthy subject. Once again, cheating isn't allowed, like designating perfectly healthy people as asymptomatic cases or carriers. Either we are trying to understand the causes of suffering, or we are not; and if a supposed unique cause does not correlate with its supposed effects, then it probably isn't the cause.

Then it would be necessary to isolate a *pure* sample of the virus and show that exposure did consistently and uniquely cause the disease, and not cause anything else. And lastly, to show that the virus is contagious, it would be necessary to extract it from a subject who had been made sick only by such exposure, purify it, and then use it to cause sickness in another healthy subject. That would have to be done by the normal means of transmission, and once again without cheating, by injecting or whatever.

Koch's Postulates, as the above tests are called, are nothing more than a systematic breakdown of the premise of viral disease, and the stages inferred that would confirm it. There is one other test that would help, or series of tests, namely, to investigate competing hypotheses alongside for comparison. But is that done? Generally not. None of those tests are, or certainly not with rigour.

In fact, proving the viral cause of an illness looks more like this. A sample of tissue is taken from a diseased subject, mashed up, diluted, sterilised, preserved with chemicals, filtered to remove lumps; and then, the resulting soup is injected straight into the brain of a monkey. When the monkey gets sick and dies, the claim is made that the virus has been purified and isolated and proven to be the distinct cause of all cases.

This method is obviously invalid in at least five ways:

1) It presupposes that the sample must contain the virus of interest.

2) The sample is very far from pure and there is very little idea of what it really contains.

3) Normal spread of illness is not even remotely theorised to involve injection into the brain, yet those are the lengths they have to go to for a reaction.

4) Injecting *anything* non-self into the brain is likely to cause severe illness.

5) Other possible candidates for cause are not explored.

But believe it or not, that is more or less how it was decided that polio paralysis is caused by a polio virus. It doesn't take a genius to see several very significant problems. Then, there are the issues of sample size, control groups, bias, and all the rest.

Things are better today, we are told. But are they? However diligent virologists may be these days, their work necessarily invokes assumptions solidified by experiments like the above. Critiques of the current state of virology are no less damning—to date, it seems no government health department in the world is owning up to having a pure sample of the SARS-CoV-2 virus [11]. That's a bit concerning, given that those same authorities claim to know everything about it, and have changed all our lives because of it.

Identification of a virus seldom seems to follow an open investigation of what makes people sick. When health authorities look for a virus, it is only a virus they find. When there are huge gaps in the description of a viral genome, they are filled by a computer algorithm and not by chemistry work. The exploration generally begins with the massive supposition that a biological agent is responsible. Any toxicologist would disagree with that reasoning, and so do I. Making it all work depends on so many fixes and fudges, from the fairly plausible, such as asymptomatic carriers, to the completely nonsensical, such as variants without symptoms, or for which there is no test, that I am very much not sold on the theory, even though for more than half my life I was.

As far as I am concerned, there is yet no solid basis for fearing any virus. I am far more fearful of misguided people in authority. The degree to which we have lost the right to act on our own beliefs is horrifying, but even worse is the degree to which we must now act on the beliefs of others.

Things have changed. At the end of the 20th century, if you told your doctor you'd caught something from a toilet seat, he might have laughed at you. Now we are supposed to believe we can die from a virus—and kill others—after sitting on a bench in an empty park. If you don't believe it, a policeman might put you in handcuffs and make you believe it.

At college, having a cold was no excuse to skip clinic: the words, "Unless you are at death's door," were used. At school, it might get us off games if we were lucky. Now it shuts down whole states and causes doctors to ex-communicate patients in need. And for what? But I have never, as far as I can tell, caught anything from a patient. I still get colds and flu, thank God, but according to other patterns of which I am now more aware.

I have treated people with shingles and not ended up with blisters, although for some reason this illness is not known to be contagious, even though it involves a contagious virus. And I must have handled thousands of pairs of feet with verrucas and warts, yet my hands are not covered in verrucas and warts. I did once treat somebody who was going bald, and now I am going bald, so I could be wrong.

Basic diagnostic theory tells us that one sign doesn't make a pathology. Therefore, labelling symptomless people as sick based only on a single, shoddy test for an unproven entity could fairly be described as fraud and medical malpractice. Two tests for the same sign still amount to one sign, no pathology. And the belief that every symptom or sniffle is a danger that, unless checked, will lead to a cascade of serious problems is just outright false. Who benefits from these distortions? Not patients.

Whether or not the existence of viral disease has been settled, what should really concern us is something else: *susceptibility*. If polio really is a dangerous virus, why is it only dangerous to about 1% of people who get it? Why are measles only dangerous in Africa? Why do millions of Australians get bitten by mosquitoes every single day, but only a handful develop joint pain and fever? How can one person living in a city centre hostel during a flu outbreak be fine, while a shepherd living on a remote hillside gets flu and dies? Aren't these questions of far greater importance than how to wipe every virus off the face of the earth? I think so.

Doctors and scientists ought really to be interested in why only some people succumb to these illnesses, instead of just which toxic chemicals might stop it.

The answer to disease lies in health, and stresses of one kind or another are the only areas worthy of our attention if we are serious about it. Toxicity is one major cause of stress, and one of the effects is to disturb regulation. And regulation is central to the issue of why the body sometimes seems to go wrong.

What are thought to be viruses will always be with us, and they can always be found in sick people, since the breakdown of cells is part of life. Whether we call it a virus, or an exosome, or simply biological garbage and cellular debris, naming it is a far cry from saying it is the problem, or that destroying it is the way to secure health. Even the most avid adherents to the viral theory ought still to admit they are looking in completely the wrong place for practical solutions. Whatever we choose to believe about viral illness, the question of what we can do about it still leads us back to the toxic state sooner or later.

The good news is that our bodies detox all the time. Our main task as patients is simply to allow or enable it through reasonably careful living, and as practitioners, by helping to keep everything working as it should. Forcible detoxification is seldom a good idea except in particular circumstances, and this should generally only be undertaken with expert guidance. Health-based measures of any kind can encourage natural detoxification to accelerate spontaneously, sometimes leading to a healing crisis. Therefore, that is a strong reason for assessing the toxic state of the individual to some extent, even if we think of our treatment as merely a specialism.

When actively trying to reduce toxins in the body, the most important task is therefore to remove the source. Most of us can afford to clean up our lifestyles and improve the quality of our diets, and in the majority of cases, not much else is needed. A detox on the home, the office, the car, and the food cupboards can bring bigger dividends than going straight for the body.

And not all toxins are chemical. A mobile phone mast or power lines close to home can cause all kinds of problems. Situations and occupations can be toxic or even caustic, and many people have found their health improve from a change of job, or release from some kind of personal bind. There are toxic personalities also. A great resource here is David Gillespie's life-changing *Taming Toxic People* [12].

Any sources embedded in the body need particular attention, and one important suspect there is dental work. Metal fillings do more than just supply mercury, they also cause strange electrical effects. Root canal fillings can be a health disaster [13]: they do not 'save' a tooth, they mummify a dead tooth and maintain its presence in the body. Once there, having them extracted can be a big deal as well—not something to be rushed into.

Teeth may also have a role in detoxification. We can pack toxins into a tooth, the tooth goes rotten and falls out, and we carry on with our lives. It is commonly understood that keeping our teeth in good order helps keep our bodies in good order. But fewer recognise that keeping our bodies in order is what keeps our teeth in good order.

The historical reasons for mercury in dentistry may go beyond its usefulness as a packing material. Mercury was commonly used in medicine at one point, because its extreme toxicity also gave it some useful properties as a suppressant. It was seen as a cure, since it could make a rash disappear. In fact, it was still present in topical (skin) treatments right up to the 1970s, and in some countries, it still is. A rash appears whenever the skin is trying to get rid of something. Topical mercury is a far greater threat than whatever the skin is trying to get rid of, and so the outflow shuts down for protection. The skin seals itself up: it appears to heal, until the mercury has gone away, that is.

However, the trouble with this approach is twofold. Firstly, the problem is internalised: the glowing complexion belies the disease beneath. And secondly, the mercury itself is fearsomely dangerous.

Modern skin treatments work by a similar principle, albeit with less obvious risks. Steroids and other topical creams likewise cause a reversal of the outflow of waste, but the trouble is the waste then isn't removed and repeat application is needed. Eventually, more severe systemic disease can appear, such as asthma.

Milder 'emollients' are mainly petroleum-based, and the subtle irritation they cause has a similar effect. At first the soft, moist cream seems to soothe, but then after a few hours or days, the irritation has built up until further application is needed.

Mineral-oil based moisturisers and lip-balms do the same thing, leading to endless repeat applications and dependency. Hence, there are plenty of people who dare not leave the house without the comforting feel of a lip-balm in their pocket, or a bottle of some lotion in their handbag.

The way to reverse this dependency includes switching to a 100% natural product with no chemical additives whatsoever. Sometimes the switch is enough. But it can also be necessary to deal with why there was an irritation in the first place. In severe cases of dermatitis, it might not be so simple.

Extending this understanding to dentistry, assuming the body may use a tooth as a dumping ground for toxins, one can speculate that someone once thought packing a tooth might be a permanent solution, not just for filling but for suppressing the actual process of tooth decay. Perhaps somebody out there knows and can tell me ...

It really does matter whether so-called contagious microbial illnesses really are caused by microbes, or whether the microbes just show up and add to our woes—or if they are in fact the body's normal and healthy response to toxicity or some other change (more on that idea later). It may be different in each case. But if we have got this wrong, then not only would the causes of disease have been wrongly attributed, the solutions would have been expensive and dangerous failures as well. The result would be incalculable human suffering and a monumental waste of effort. The only way to know might be to address the toxic state, and then see what is left, in each and every case. Therefore, this has to be at least one of our top priorities as healers. As to why it might be of particular interest to osteopaths; the answer lies in the relationship between body structure and natural immunity.

There are several pieces to the puzzle still to be covered later.

In recent years, our healing processes have been positively weaponised against us. Since 2020, those who have exhibited even mild symptoms have been isolated, and in some cases put on excessive medical treatment, supposedly to protect the rest of us, when most of us never asked for such protection to begin with. Demanding everybody places the welfare of unnamed others ahead of their own welfare leaves everybody's welfare suppressed, as we have seen.

We each have our own set of risks in life to balance out. Those who fear germs the most, and those who fear most for their livelihoods, can all act accordingly. It is up to each of us. But I would suggest that those most panicky about illness should not think of pursuing a career in public health, for all our sakes.

This so-called protection has led to the most widespread abuse of human rights most of us have ever witnessed, including, huge restrictions on lawful activity, registration with the authorities to buy food, and the blanket coercion of healthy people to receive medical treatment lacking any long-term safety data. Perfectly healthy people were punished for going about their business and, unlawfully imprisoned in their own homes [14]. Citizens were obliged to police each other, and the degree to which many went along with this is chilling. Decency was criminalised. Dissent was silenced. And doctors threw ethical norms out of the window, usually without a whimper of protest.

Whom exactly this is supposed to have saved is unclear. But it is very clear whom it has benefitted. It has led to the greatest upwards wealth transfer in history [15]. And the scope for state interference in ordinary people's lives has been ratcheted up several notches. Were there political and economic motivations that could have shaped events negatively? Obviously, there were.

Within a toxicity-centred paradigm for disease, none of this could have happened. Germ theory is not only crucial to the suppression of natural therapy and the promotion of harmful chemicals. It is also a prop for some quite major political choices that can't be justified without it. If germ theory goes, then whole power structures would fall, but the ordinary person would be far better off in so many ways. It's easy to see why there is so much effort in keeping it alive.

[1] Brent Leung, Film, *House of Numbers*, 2009, https://www.houseofnumbers.com/.

[2] Simon Oxenham, *Why do we fall for false positives even though they're common?* New Scientist 8 Aug 2016 https://www.newscientist.com/article/2100273-why-do-we-fall-for-false-positives-even-though-theyre-common/.

[3] Bill Bryson, book, *A Short History of Nearly Everything*.

[4] Hoyle F, Wickramasinghe NC. *Influenza – Evidence against Contagion: Discussion Paper.* Journal of the Royal Society of Medicine. 1990;83(4):258-261. doi:10.1177/014107689008300417.

[5] World Health Organisation, *Measles*, https://www.who.int/en/news-room/fact-sheets/detail/measles.

[6] Centres for Disease Control, *Measles Cases and Outbreaks*, https://www.cdc.gov/measles/data-research/index.html.

[7] Jayne Donegan, *Measles outbreaks: the song remains the same*, https://www.jayne-donegan.co.uk/measles-outbreaks/.

[8] NIHCE Guidelines, *How should I diagnose measles?*, https://cks. nice.org.uk/topics/measles/diagnosis/clinical-diagnosis/.

[9] Janine Roberts, book, *Fear of the Invisible*.

[10] Torsten Engelbrecht and Claus Köhnlein, book, *Virus Mania*.

[11] Christine Massey, *The Identity of the Virus: Health/ Science Institutions Worldwide "Have No Record" of SARS-COV-2 Isolation/Purification*, Global Research, 16 Oct 2023, https://www.globalresearch. ca/foi-reveal-health-science-institutions-around-world-have-no-record-sars-cov-2-isolation-purification-anywhere-ever/5751969.

[12] David Gillespie, book, *Taming Toxic People*.

[13] Hal Huggins, *Root Canal Dangers*, Weston A Price Foundation, https://www.westonaprice.org/health-topics/dentistry/ root-canal-dangers/.

[14] Victorian Ombudsman, *Tower lockdown breached human rights, Ombudsman finds*, https://www.ombudsman.vic.gov.au/our-impact/ news/public-housing-tower-lockdown/.

[15] Oxfam, *Ten richest men double their fortunes in pandemic while incomes of 99 percent of humanity fall*, Press Release 17 January 2022, https://www.oxfam.org/en/press-releases/ten-richest-men-double-their-fortunes-pandemic-while-incomes-99-percent-humanity.

Missing Link 6:
Structural adjustment

He calls himself Mr. because he has not
acquired the privilege of giving a certificate
when a patient dies on his hands.

—Mark Twain (giving testimony in support of
osteopaths)

When Dr Andrew Taylor Still introduced his theory of osteopathy to the world in the 1870s, he had no desire to complement medicine or fill in its gaps. His view was that medicine was a colossal failure, and his intention was to replace it with something altogether better. In many ways that need hasn't gone away, it's just that medicine has acquired so much power that its current hegemony can't be challenged. Were it not for politics and huge commercial power imbalances, that might not be the case.

Still's idea of looking to the physical structure of the spine and the posture to improve general health was not new. Some natural therapists of the 19th century understood that diet, exercise, hydrotherapy, homoeopathy, herbs, and so on were not enough, and that chemical and energetic interventions also required good physical adjustment. They recognised that a good diet alone couldn't make you healthy if your body couldn't process nutrients; that the spine was involved, not just the guts; and that a rounded healing system needed to take that into account. They were keen to learn from the body adjusters and bonesetters, who found pleasing results in general health from addressing the physical structure.

Dr Still's theory was that the mechanics of the spine, ribs, and other structures were crucial to the distribution of blood, and that where blood went, health would follow. That these ideas have gone out of vogue has nothing to do with whether or not they worked, and everything to do with the active memory-holing of anything truly potent that leads away from drugs.

As much as early osteopaths drew upon the ideas of other natural therapies, it was mostly to do with ensuring a background adequacy of basic needs. It wasn't about seeking *other techniques* to address *other parts* of the body. Their system was already complete.

Nowadays, when nutritionists, homoeopaths, herbalists, and others look to structural 'adjuncts' to complete the picture, including what is known today as osteopathy, they are not really seeing it as an important way to support the organs. They usually see it as a way to address regions and systems of the body where they have little direct reach. They talk about modalities for this and modalities for that. Very few realise today that osteopathy was conceived as a stand-alone therapy that was so broad it could manage pretty well on its own.

In that sense, osteopathy, as practised these days by only a very few, is one of the only therapies I can think of that comes close to holism. Many others do aim for it, including some modern osteopaths; but if they employ nutrition, needles, cranial, visceral massage, psychotherapy, etcetera, as treatments for the function, and regard structural adjustment as something 'to address the structural aspects', then they have missed the point of holism.

It's a shame, because there is so much potential in these tools when a truly holistic blueprint is employed. While our modern training certainly included traditional osteopathic principles, they were dealt with largely as a matter of historic or academic interest. They weren't taught as a way to gain a clear handle on what to do in practice. And when it came to real cases, we were pretty much required to leave those ideas at the clinic door on the way in.

It is true that a good diet is necessary for good health, but it is debatable whether an aggressive dietary programme is, since a healthy body can generally sort things out given enough basic resources. True also, early osteopaths would occasionally fast a patient, and add or limit certain foods at certain stages, but that was to support the adjustive road map and not stand outside of it. Most of us older ones remember having stomachs like furnaces when we were young, and it making little difference to our wellbeing whether we ate what our mothers cooked or threw down a Mars Bar. So, a healthy body can tolerate a pizza or a hamburger. If that becomes the mainstay, then obviously, eventually, one will end up chronically sick.

But to the osteopaths, outside of such frank lifestyle issues, the missing link was how efficiently the organs were working, so that nutrients could be ingested, digested, absorbed, transported through the blood and assimilated into tissue, and so that the waste could be got rid of efficiently. All of that, they believed, depended on good adjustment. If all is well in that sense, then there is a great deal of latitude available in the human diet.

Therapists are usually aware that the digestive and other organs can be below par, but even seasoned body workers seldom think to look to the posture for the reasons. They rely on elimination diets, colonics, herbs, megadoses of vitamins, visceral massage, adaptogens, and many more things to 'correct' the imbalance. Since that does not and cannot address the causes within the posture, but merely compensate, it does not necessarily reduce the ongoing draw-down on the patient's vitality. The slippery slope down to reductionism is obvious.

Of course, if somebody suffers a food intolerance then they have to be careful. And if they depend on higher doses of vitamins, then it is a better idea to take them than not to take them. At least they will function while they work through the problem. But when we find ourselves arguing over chickpeas versus lentils or taking handfuls of vitamins just to stay on an even keel, then clearly something else is going on. Gluten is not the cause of gluten intolerance. A diabetic who avoids sugar is still diabetic. And a good mechanic is concerned with keeping the engine properly tuned, while a bad mechanic sells you a fuel additive to stop it from misfiring.

Modern osteopaths and chiropractors alike aren't taught about *adjustment, the condition*, as in the state of structural and functional harmony. They are taught about *adjustment, the method,* as in the skill of moving bones around, also known as manipulation.

Dr Still gave us the concept of *the osteopathic lesion*; another rather vague term, but a real thing, all the same. The chiropractors have their subluxation (a misaligned bone or joint), but this is not the same. The subluxation is a very local and specific thing, and they treat it very locally and specifically. Specific adjustment is the very hallmark of chiropractic, and many osteopaths have taken that direction as well. If the vertebra is turned left, turn it back into line with a rotational adjustment the other way. Their theory is that in doing so, the disease associated with the subluxation will be removed. Being treated this way can be quite a shock to the system. It may work in practice, but I see many cases where it hasn't.

The osteopathic lesion does not mean the out-of-place bone, although a localised bony disturbance can certainly be a manifestation of the lesion. As I see it, the lesion is the entire pattern of stress and strain unique to the patient that may cause a bone to be out of place or not. The important point is that it raises stress responses, either locally or generally, above what is needed to maintain good function.

It is legitimate to talk about lesioned segments or bones. But to my mind, they are not synonymous with the lesion itself.

The big difference therefore between chiropractic and osteopathy is that the chiropractor believes you can correct the lesion by correcting the bone, while the osteopath believes that in order to correct the bone, you correct the lesion. The subluxation is an effect. But to the

chiropractors, it is causal, and presumes a level of mis-
trust in the arrangement.

I appreciate these points may not sink in at first. But
bear with me for now.

The fact is spinal segments or other bones do not simply go stiff or jump out of place for no reason. They are
acted upon by countless forces from all over the place.
Some are local, such as ligaments, muscles, and other
bones. And some are distant—whole waves of stress
throughout the spine and body. The chair, the car, the
job, the diet, the breathing, the state of the bowels, the
patient's hopes, fears, and dreams … all are present to
some extent. An indigestible meal can set up a lesion.

To straighten the bone and expect the rest of the universe to unravel around it is therefore fanciful at best. But
that is what chiropractors aim to do. This isn't what I say,
it's what they say themselves: DD Palmer's words, "Chiropractic is specific or it is nothing," hang on the walls of
their offices. This obvious appeal to reductionism sounds
good, but it's a bit like architects saying they must have
nice sharp pencils; it leaves unanswered the question of
what these tools are really for.

In the chiropractic philosophy, the bone out of place
stresses a nerve and that stresses the organ. Straighten
the bone and the healing follows. In contrast, osteopathically, the bone is neither the beginning nor end of the
causal chain, and the clicks and pops of adjustment are
therefore a possible result of change, but not the cause
of change. Making the local adjustment the object of the
exercise sets us up to fail. But out of this intention was
born the discipline of specific adjustment.

In short, making bones click is not synonymous with getting somebody better. All the same, chiropractors have remained very popular all over the world, so they must be doing something right. So, it may nevertheless be possible to use these direct and specific skills in a holistic or indirect way. I'm just not clear how.

Chiropractors might disagree with this analysis, and I hope that they would, otherwise they're in the wrong business! I'm not knocking it; if direct and linear therapy is what chiropractors believe in, then they should be proud of it. I am saying that specific adjustment sits at one end of a spectrum and stating the case for the opposite. The other end of the spectrum is called general treatment, or body adjustment, which aims to normalise the relationships between whole regions of the body at a time. I can't go into the exact techniques here: but for all sorts of reasons, which I have tried to explain, general treatment is more physiologically appropriate—usually. Occasionally, I treat specifically, but always within a context of general patterns.

Osteopaths should have no problem with these discussions, but the fact is many do.

So, if a spine is lesioned in many places with palpable disturbances from end to end, the specific adjuster would correct all the subluxations, so that in doing so, the entire pattern will reduce. I disagree. It sounds reasonable because that is how you fix a car, one piece at a time. But, in a living system, you get the whole thing working properly and then the parts can take care of themselves. This is the essence of holism, in my view, and why comparisons with car mechanics, although helpful, are limited. When one part of the spine moves, it all moves. If you twist a piece of string from both ends tighter and tighter, you get waves and kinks along the length. If you just go straight to the kinks and force them straight, you actually put more stress into the system, not less. And in health, there are consequences to taking this approach. You must untwist the entire pattern, and then the kinks will become less of an issue. You may even get larger waves as a tightly wound system relaxes. Following treatment, many patients are surprised that they can feel more wonky for a while yet have less pain and greater freedom of movement.

These principles aren't limited to painful kinks in the spine; patterns of stress pass through and in between every system of the body. Some of this is fairly abstract. But importantly, there is no absolute demarcation between soma and viscera—container and contents. Many of these relationships are reciprocal. Every part of the body, in as much as there are parts, is self-maintaining, self-regulating, self-repairing. But to function well, a part needs support from the entire system. If an organ is misfiring in some way, it is not the organ that needs correction, it is the system that needs adjusting. If you ignore the global situation, the organ will never cope, no matter how expertly you treat it directly.

The spine is particularly relevant in terms of the tuning of the system, because a disordered spine must rob resources from corresponding organs to deal with the extra workload of resisting gravity and avoiding collapse. But there is more to it, because when the spine is disturbed, regulation itself will be upset.

Furthermore, there are various multiplier effects, which means that quite a small disturbance to posture can result in a major disturbance to regulation. The precise mechanisms don't really matter for this discussion, but this is the basic outline of the osteopathic lesion idea, as I see it.

Don't repeat any of this in college though, or you may fail! But it has all been confirmed by much rigorous investigation. And by now, it should be obvious that you can't treat the spine simply as a number of independent segments, nor treat any system or organ as if isolated or independent.

The concepts of the osteopathic lesion and body adjustment are not merely hypothetical. The early osteopaths' accomplishments in all areas of disease are documented, and in everything from infectious diseases to reproductive problems, they were once a perfectly sound choice of physician for any patient. During the Spanish Flu, they had a batting average that makes you wonder what on earth the medical doctors were playing at.

They weren't doing visceral massage as such, or dry needling, or functional medicine, or treating the cranial rhythm. They used postural adjustment and good health management.

Back pain is mentioned in the old texts, but not so much as a condition in its own right. If they treated the patient, not the condition, the associated symptoms went away, including the back pain. Sports injuries weren't really a separate problem: they were just injuries. The big difference with a sports injury is that the patient wants to go and do it again.

It was politics and commercial pragmatics that removed these ideas from our medical lexicon, not lack of effectiveness. Osteopathy was turned into a theory of musculoskeletal therapy based largely around medical orthopaedics and physiotherapy, with some low-key extensions into other areas. As such, the field is now seen as a specialism based on certain techniques and certain systems of the body, rather than as a unifying theory of health and disease.

Some modern critiques of the structural lesion try to drive us further away from holism, creating overly detailed pastiches for the lesion theory in order to knock them down. They ask too much of the lesion, as if it were the route to a precise curative, rather than more accurately as a vital and often elusive link in the chain.

Fryer 2016 [1] goes to great lengths to argue why the osteopathic lesion (AKA somatic dysfunction) is an outdated idea, but then, bizarrely, posits an impressively detailed and well-reasoned explanation for it. It isn't light reading, and in my opinion, it isn't complete or entirely correct; not least since it is still seeing the disease rather than the health. Nevertheless, it is a worthy attempt to flesh out the mechanisms involved.

Fryer's main objections relate not to actual physiology, but to variability of mechanism, inconsistency of diagnosis, and difficulty communicating amongst practitioners and with other professions—politics and practicalities, essentially.

Why that means we have to abandon a priceless discovery is beyond me. If anything, the study exemplifies the folly of a reductionist approach, the very thing researchers have done their best to promote through research of this kind.

It is fair to say that the lesion idea is poorly understood. Nevertheless, it is not without considerable empirical truth. For example, cardiovascular events are objectively associated with lesion features [2]. The mechanisms involved may be far more complicated and varied than the early osteopaths expected. All the same, we witness things ascribed to the lesion, sometimes when there is no other manageable explanation. If scientists take a dog apart looking for the bark, they've only themselves to blame when they can't find it. And if professionals in other disciplines fail to grasp biological reality, then that is their problem.

A neutral position might be that we need a modern explanation to work on, rather than taking a century-old definition and throwing it out altogether. But the awkward reality is that the early osteopaths did just fine.

I suppose adjustment and lesioning are really semantic opposites. Things are either in adjustment, or in lesion, or in degrees of both. The debate should be about what it means in practice. Examining broad and subjective ideas with too high a magnification is one way to deny their importance, and this is something we need to guard against in all areas of life.

Personally speaking, I am sold, and my flag is nailed to the mast. My proposal is that we scrap the need to get ever more specific, and instead paint in much broader brushstrokes, so that in order to be effective, we won't need a radiology suite and pathology lab in every clinic. How we

1,240 CASES TREATED WITHOUT DRUGS.
WASHINGTON INSTITUTE OF OSTEOPATHY.

DISEASES TREATED.	No. of Cases Treated	No. of Cases Cured	No. of Cases Greatly Benefited	No. of Cases Benefited	Cases Not Benefited	No. of Cases Without Fair Trial	Average No. of Treatments
Stomach Troubles, Gastralgia, Indigestion, Gastritis, etc	148	64	51	22	6	5	15
Constipation, from a few months to 25 years' standing	89	54	23	5	4	3	17
Rheumatism, Muscular, Gouty, Articular, etc.	90	21	35	23	7	4	22
Sciatica, Sciatic Rheumatism, Neuralgia, etc	27	16	5	1	2	3	14
Lumbago, Lumb Sprain, and Neuralgia	39	31	4	2	..	2	12
Neurasthenia, Nervous Prostration, etc	59	26	20	9	3	1	19
Spinal Irritation	14	3	6	2	2	1	17
Spinal Curvature	17	8	1	5	2	1	33
Other Spinal Troubles, Neuralgias and Weakness	38	17	12	7	1	1	29
Female Troubles, Menstrual, Uterine and Ovarian	154	54	50	36	6	8	15
Neuralgia, Trigeminal, Cranial and Intercostal	78	41	20	10	5	2	18
Chronic Headache, from Causes Other Than Neuralgia	16	10	5	1	..	..	18
Chronic Catarrh	23	5	13	2	2	1	17
Eye and Ear Troubles	53	12	12	11	12	6	16
Kidneys and Bladder, Albuminuria, Diabetes, Cystitis	17	5	5	3	2	2	16
Epileptic Convulsions and Other Fits	15	2	2	2	9	..	26
Liver Troubles	9	2	5	1	..	1	22
Heart Troubles, Functional Derangements	14	4	3	3	3	1	18
Rectal Troubles, Piles, Rectalgia, Rectocele	12	6	3	1	2	..	14
Joint Trouble, Hip Disease, Adhesions and Synovitis	26	7	10	6	2	1	25
Sprains and Dislocations, Knee, Hip, Ankle, Elbow, Shoulder	43	20	14	6	2	1	22
General Debility	25	5	13	5	1	1	22
Paralysis, Hemiplegia, General and Local	52	8	13	22	8	1	24
Asthma	24	6	12	2	4	..	21
Varicose Veins, Including Varicose Ulcers	9	2	3	3	..	1	20
Locomotor Ataxia	7	..	3	2	1	1	19
Enlarged Tonsils and Chronic Tonsilitis	7	3	1	3	..	..	13
Insomnia	10	5	3	2	..	..	12
Intestinal Troubles, Appendicitis, Chronic Diarrhoea	15	7	2	4	1	1	20
Lung and Throat Troubles, Including Chronic Bronchitis	36	13	9	8	5	1	16
Goitre	13	3	4	5	1	..	23
Acute Cases, Fevers, LaGrippe and Colds	26	22	2	2	..	..	5
Miscellaneous Cases *	35	16	12	2	4	1	16
TOTALS	1,240	498	376	218	97	51	616

No drugs required—what osteopaths were treating with enviable success at the start of the 20th century. Cases were recorded by the Washington Institute of Osteopathy, Seattle, from June 10, 1898 to May 1, 1902. Various digestive problems made up the biggest area of work. What are now called musculoskeletal cases were less than a quarter of the total. See also listed asthma, eczema, epilepsy, breast cancer, prostate troubles, insomnia, paralysis, and many gynaecological cases. From the Journal *The Osteopathic World*, edited by JM Littlejohn. Courtesy of the Institute of Classical Osteopathy.

do this in practice needs different thinking tools—take a step back in time, in other words—hence this book.

Having established that there is a level of truth to the structural lesion, let's not rip the circuitry out of the black box, but rather, let's accept there is a great deal we won't ever understand about the intelligence of the body, and deal with it respectfully.

Alas, the very term 'osteopathy' invites confusion, since the intention was as much about blood as bones. Dr Still and others were not treating structural problems as such, but rather using structure as a handle on the deeper organic physiology. If it sounds far-fetched, remember that this was bread and butter for practitioners who depended on results.

Once the Flexner Report had done its worst, osteopathy, as Still envisaged it, was dying in the USA. His protégé, John Martin Littlejohn, brought it to England to save it, and founded the first major school outside America.

By the time Littlejohn died, there was much pressure to reform in England, too. The old ideas got thrown out; they literally purged the libraries of old texts at one point, and the medicalisation of the field accelerated after the Second World War. It has remained acceptable to talk about the *viscero-somatic reflex*—the influence of the organs on the musculoskeletal system—since medicine still needs to explain the referred pain of angina or gallstones somehow. But the opposite—the *somato-visceral reflex*—is medically inconvenient and has been shelved along with the osteopathic lesion. Hence, general health theory among osteopaths today is now skewed towards the fluid, cellular and chemical aspects—things beyond the musculoskeletal realm in a reductionist paradigm—and thereby rendered somewhat off-label to the general structural practitioner.

By the time of Littlejohn's death, the profession had dug so deeply into the minutiae of the physiology that they began to lose Still's sense of how it all fitted together. Osteopathy would have gone away completely except in name, were it not for a gentleman named John Wernham, who had been Littlejohn's neighbour as a boy and later trained under him. Wernham rejected the later reforms and stayed well away from the stifling new regulatory framework up until his death in 2007, aged 99, still practising and lecturing right up to the end.

Wernham's genius was to take what Littlejohn and others had pulled apart and put it all back together again. In doing so, he made it better, easier to do, safer, more effective, and more universally applicable than ever before. But by then, much of the profession had turned their backs on this work, and some now treat Wernham's name as a joke. Nevertheless, many lean on his trademark, Classical Osteopathy, sometimes offering it as a minor modality within their overall repertoires. Others avoid it altogether, saying Wernham was old-fashioned or out of touch. Such is the luck of those who are way ahead of their time.

Most of all, Wernham kept osteopathy utterly true to the original intent of the discipline, which made his work threatening to the modern eclectic styles. In turn, one might suppose that modern cranial, visceral, and musculoskeletal osteopathy might have been allowed to persist because they are not a threat to the medical establishment.

I was lucky enough to meet Mr Wernham, not long before his passing. He was scathing about the modern colleges and instantly abrasive towards those of us who trained in them.

The number of practitioners in the world today who truly took on board Wenham's approach, and haven't messed it up by using it as just another modality, might fit in the proverbial London Taxi, or perhaps a tube train carriage. And you probably won't have heard of them, since it's not a way to become rich and famous when the zeitgeist now favours reductionism, eclecticism, and multiple modalities of linear treatment, in place of true holism.

Structural adjustment aside, the choice to embrace holism requires a decisive shift of priorities in any branch of healing. One learns that to get where you want to go, you sometimes have to take the long way around. Once there is some grasp of the distinction between true holism and simply doing lots of different things to the patient, then some discussion of complex systems behaviour needs to take place. Read on.

[1] Fryer G, *Somatic dysfunction: An osteopathic conundrum*, International Journal of Osteopathic Medicine (2016), http://dx.doi.org/10.1016/j.ijosm.2016.02.002.

[2] Nicholas A S, DeBias D A, Ehrenfeuchter W, England K M, England R W, Greene C H et al., *A somatic component to myocardial infarction*. Br Med J (Clin Res Ed) 1985; 291 :13 doi:10.1136/bmj.291.6487.13.

Missing Link 7:
Chaos—complexity
and non-linearity

*It is utterly implausible that a mathematical formula should
make the future known to us, and those who think it can
would once have believed in witchcraft.*

—Jacob Bernoulli

The mainstream osteopathic profession always saw John Wernham (previous chapter) as an outlier and found it very difficult to relate to his theories. There were many who admired him but failed to grasp the essence of the extraordinarily elegant framework he developed. And there were those who disagreed strongly with it because it didn't connect with the clinical physiology they understood. There were those who followed in his footsteps and could sort of see where he was going, but lacked the spirit needed to follow him there with commitment.

However, there are a few who took it in and held it right down in their soul, and I have been lucky enough to know one or two of them; they are a small and very special group of practitioners. You won't see them present their work in a 5,000-seat arena. They go about it

unnoticed, because there is seldom a whizz-bang epiph-
any or earth-shattering breakthrough except in the most
superficial of cases. It is in the complex and chronic cases
where the patient's life and health just return fairly qui-
etly to stability, almost without anyone realising it is happening. So, it would all be completely unimpressive, but
for the fact that hardly anybody else is really achieving it
with the same consistency. Nor are they doing it in a way
that involves down-to-earth, kitchen sink practical methods we can demonstrate and teach and apply on a desert
island if we have to. The results are easily dismissed as
purely spontaneous recovery. I mean, if a natural healer
could clear the problem, it can't have been that bad, right?
Except that these are often the cases that have defeated
every other practitioner.

There are plenty of claims for both mystics and
healthcare experts alike. And whether they really stack
up in terms of our broader outcome measures is highly
doubtful; but whether or not they do, neither group can
make accessible what they do. There is nothing democratic in either modern medicine or the more highly esoteric alternatives.

Wernham was not asking his students to hold any
occult or esoteric knowledge; he was merely asking them
to be good craftsmen and trust the ability of the human
body to heal. In that sense, he was continuing an ages old
tradition of healing that you have to work in practical,
creative, subtle, and often indirect ways, because you cannot engage with a complex system in a direct and specific
way and get precisely what you want every time. Complex systems do not ever behave entirely as we expect.

There is always some departure that makes repeatability impossible. Most of us fight against that, but Wernham leveraged it.

While Wernham was often accused of being an outlier with strange theories, it was in fact the mainstream osteopaths, not Wernham, who took the field in a new direction. His work was a challenge to the highly linear direction of medicine that the modern osteopaths began falling over themselves to emulate. He was originally a war photographer, at a time when good photography demanded both an engineer's skill and a worthy artistic vision—you need both to be a craftsman.

During the same period when Wernham was developing his ideas, the field of 'Chaos' was emerging out of the hard sciences as, among other things, a way to tackle unpredictability in nature. Wernham may not have known much about it, but he was also recognising and dealing with the problems of complexity and non-repeatability in his own way.

Chaos is not really a theory, but a collection of theories all to do with the real-world behaviour of complex systems, something that was actively avoided before digital computers appeared, because there was simply no way to solve the mathematics. The only way to get answers in complexity is by performing vast numbers of calculations, one after the other, each one beginning with the output of the one before. And since there can never be enough calculations, nor enough measurements to make them all, there is always an error. And the longer we run our simulations, the bigger the errors become, until the results unavoidably attain uselessness, sooner or later. If we can use more calculations to slice our subject smaller and smaller, we can get better answers over short periods *if* all the right assumptions are included in the model. We can just as easily get wrong answers ... only faster.

Only since the 1980s has huge enough processing power been available to make chaos accessible academically and its importance viscerally obvious to the masses. Until then, human understanding of complexity required an acceptance that there is a lot of confusion and unpredictability in the universe.

For aeons, we have used other tools to deal with it, and the atheists like nothing more than to diminish those tools, even though they can't deny them to be the highly developed products of our natural evolution.

In engineering, the practical approach was to keep everything well within parameters of stability in order to avoid catastrophe. This, in turn, deprived scientists of a solid handle on the richness of emergent behaviour available in complex systems, if only we could tame it enough to tap into it without blowing ourselves to pieces. What engineering really struggled with and therefore actively avoided before the late 20th century was un-stability. And modern medicine is an extension of engineering, not of philosophy.

When Andrew Taylor Still first came up with his osteopathy, he may have been working in a fairly direct way. His exceptional talent seems to have been in knowing precisely where to kick the machine to get it to start.

In healing, where and how hard to 'kick' is different every time, even in two similar cases. And a deep understanding of philosophy, religion and history fed this extraordinary intuition of Still's, as well as the sciences. This made it fairly unrepeatable in the modern scientific sense.

Dr Still urged studies of the philosophy of medicine above its techniques, and it is likely that his graduates were better in some ways after six months of training than modern graduates with a five- or six-year Masters Degree. After all, we would not have those degrees today had the early results not been deeply impressive. In a day's work, practitioners would tackle cases their modern counterparts are taught to refer onwards automatically.

The 20th century efforts to inject repeatability involved osteopaths going deeper and deeper into the scientific minutiae, as an engineer would. After 100 years, what they failed to deliver was any kind of practical, teachable system. And the repeatability simply wasn't there.

Practitioners today reject their work, not because the science was invalid—it wasn't—but because after all that research it still didn't lead to consistent prescriptions. Their inability to translate the long lists of lesions and detailed diagrams of bodily reflexes into a practical therapy was the obstacle. But the modern profession wrongly assumes it was the original osteopathic premise that had failed and have done their best to erase it.

Wernham's brilliance was to create a structured framework that could be taught to anyone with an open mind. It could both be true to explicable scientific reality and invoke Still's osteopathic philosophy at the same time, and could be used to deliver consistently excellent results.

It was therefore Wernham who developed osteopathy along its natural path, and the modern profession that has deviated. A lot of confusion may have arisen from calling it 'Classical Osteopathy', since the word 'classical' these days can imply linear thinking, academic formality and intolerance of novelty, rather than the beautifully elegant humane creations that are the true fruits of intellectual mastery. If the term has been misunderstood, then that is just part of the curse of osteopathy.

It is the pathology-focused direction of development by engineers that has kept medicine and all its offshoots back in the steam age. By approaching complex systems primarily from a standpoint of incredible mechanistic detail, albeit with impressive technology to draw upon, it is medicine that has got completely lost. The early natural healers were never lost, because they embraced philosophy as the guide, and science as the tool.

An in-depth understanding of chaos theories isn't necessary or even within reach for most of us. But a grasp of some of the essential concepts helps us to differentiate between a direct (linear) and indirect (non-linear) approach and see why that matters so much.

An indirect approach does not simply mean influencing problem areas from a distance, like wiggling a hip joint from the foot. It means considering elements of the situation that may not be obviously connected to the presenting problem, but which are relevant to enabling the innate intelligence of the body to solving it.

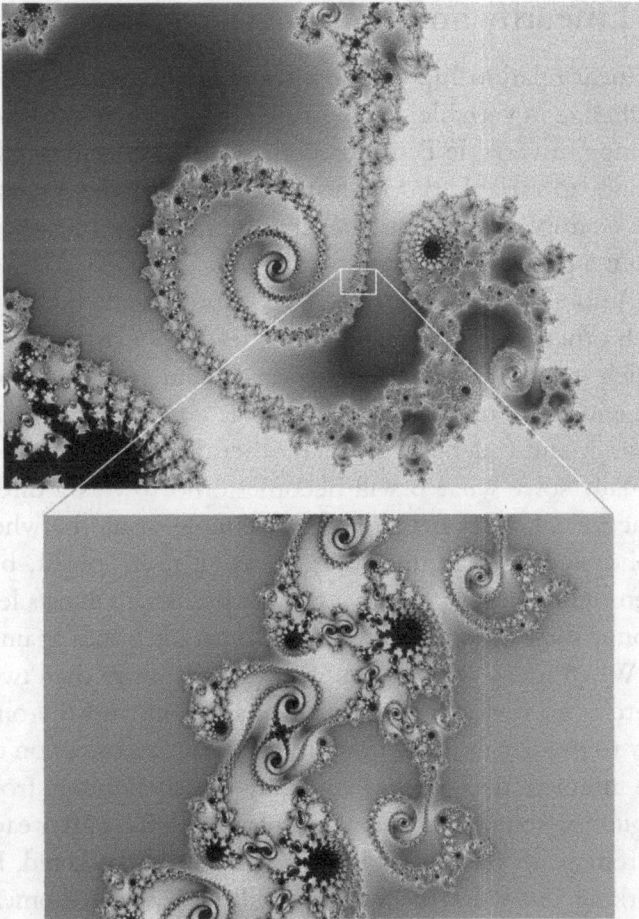

Worlds within worlds, a finite area enclosed by an infinite boundary, limitless detail derived from a limited set of rules—the Mandelbrot Set is one of the most well-known fractals. The closer we look, the more detail we see. Awe inspiring and sometimes deeply unsettling, fractals can offer important clues about nature. Reproduced from the Mandelbrot Set explorer at https://mandelbrot-set.io/ courtesy of Sebastian Eck.

1) Linearity and non-linearity

A linear relationship can be plotted as a line on a graph. A change in variable A will bring about a corresponding change in variable B that is consistent. Importantly, the change in variable B does not influence variable A again. An example might be the change in mass or weight when a glass is filled with water.

A non-linear relationship is where both A and B change each other, so that a change in A, leads to a change in B, which leads to another change in A, and so on, making the end result much harder to calculate in advance. Thus, while A and B depend on each other directly, you cannot actually solve what B will become tomorrow as a direct function of what A is now. An example would be when a shopkeeper puts up prices to make more profit, but then the higher prices drive down sales, so he makes less money than expected and has to adjust his prices again.

When more variables interact (usually more than two) there is no possible mathematical solution, and the only way to predict the final outcome is to run a simulation of the interaction as a series of many tiny increments from beginning to end, and then, calculate the effect after each increment in turn. This is how weather is predicted, by working out what the weather will be a short moment from now, then using that result to work out what the weather will be a short moment after that, and so on. As time goes by, the calculated weather becomes further and further away from the actual weather as the errors mount up. The examples of non-linearity in, say, economics, are endless.

Instead of filling a glass with water and measuring its weight, a non-linear relationship would be where we drink a glass of water and measure our own weight. As we put more water in, our weight increases for a time, but then the rate at which our kidneys remove it changes, so that the amount we put in is not the same as the amount we retain. The number of parameters to take into account is unfathomable.

2) Complex systems

Complex systems do not have to be complicated, in the sense of having many parts, although many are. What defines them is non-linearity, and through that, complexity of behaviour. A watch has many working parts, but it is not a complex system, since each of the parts behaves in a consistent and predictable way, so the behaviour of the whole device is predictable. It is designed that way, and that's why we can rely on a watch to tell us the time.

A complex system can have few elements, but they all interact in a non-linear way. A watch designed that way would not keep steady time. As it happens, there may be non-linear interactions inside a watch, and in fact, there are. But a well-designed watch has features that isolate or govern non-linear effects, so that they do not spread outwards to affect its overall performance. In reality, non-linearity is unavoidable, it's just that engineers do their best to design it out. But this fact means we can only build devices that perform well under clearly defined sets of conditions.

In practice, non-linear complex systems do generally consist of many variables. In the drinking example above, the intensity of our thirst signal changes, and the factors that influence it are many, so that the rate at which we desire to drink water adjusts with time. In fact, every cell in our bodies changes pretty much instantly when we drink a glass of water. And both thirst and filtering in the kidneys are far more than passive effects.

There are various known regulatory systems working to keep our internal fluid levels within a fairly narrow range, and all work as matters of negative feedback—the further we get from ideal, the harder the body will work to resist that change. We may drink a precise amount of water, but there is no way to predict the precise change in our weight an hour later, not to the nearest gram. What we can reasonably expect is that over hours and days, the weight of water within us will stay more or less the same.

It is negative feedback that keeps things within the survivable range thus, and positive feedback, when it occurs, that sends them zooming off towards an extreme.

Living systems are truly non-linear. And as well as many passive homoeostatic features, there are other, more active regulatory features that can adjust the passive regulation as needed. These mechanisms are only compartmentalised to an extent. There are certain centres and organs devoted to regulation, but homoeostasis of everything is woven intricately into everything. This gives us living beings an ability to perform in an efficient and consistent way even when under a great deal of stress, when a watch, for instance, would lose time or pack up altogether.

When our internal or external circumstances go wildly out of what is typical, our bodies will then sometimes do wild things, sacrificing apparent normality in one area to maintain normality elsewhere. This does not mean that homoeostasis is failing, although we may get closer to failure during those times and will be increasingly vulnerable to additional stress.

Importantly, we may not see the stress that an organ is under: we see the changes elsewhere that the body makes to protect it. For example, osteoporosis is a change in the bone, but the problem it solves for the body is the far more immediate one of blood chemistry. The pH of the blood stays nicely neutral, so there is nothing to see there, but the body is having to scavenge bone mineral to keep it that way. We can choose to view osteoporosis as bone disease, or as blood homoeostasis, or as a survival mechanism.

Complex self-regulating systems exhibit negative feedback while within certain limits, and positive feedback when they go outside those limits. Thus, we are not stable in the way that a rock is stable. We exhibit dynamic stability the way a bicycle does. A bicycle does not go in a straight line. It proceeds in a series of small wobbles. And through the design of the bicycle, a wobble to the left automatically induces a wobble to the right to counter it. This is passive negative feedback in the system. The wavy path a bike makes is not regular and repeating; it varies the entire time. If it veers suddenly to avoid a pothole, the deviation may be too great for the bike to counter passively, and so, positive feedback threatens to tip the bike over. To counter this, the rider will have to do something more physical to bring it back into line. The system may go through a series of wild sways before it returns to full control. The input of the rider is a sort of uber homoeostatic mechanism doing extraordinary things at an extraordinary time. But it is still negative feedback, this time involving the trained brain of the rider. If he fails to keep things under control, positive feedback overwhelms the system, and he falls off.

Health could be likened to the bike moving along normally under passive dynamic stability, and the expression of symptoms—often called illness—might be seen as the more drastic deviations to avoid the pothole. If there were a therapist in this arrangement, their job would be to allow the bike and rider to maintain their own stability but be ready to give a helping shove from the outside if needed. This seems to be what Still was good at. Importantly, the shove must be carefully placed and timed, since it could just as easily make matters worse.

Obviously, some riders take a more bumpy road than others, and ride it harder. Their stability is more precarious and takes more energy to maintain.

Curiously, a look in a medical physiology textbook suggests that normal physiology 'just is' and remains the same, no matter the shape of the road. It stays like that until pathology strikes, which it seems to do for no reason. There is no pothole, the rider is in perfect control, but the bike just flips. At that stage, the body's natural response is to take drugs. That is generally how medical physiology and pathology are laid out. Things do need understanding at that level, but what also needs to be understood and investigated are the conditions that lead up to making the bike flip. By whizzing right past that part, medicine generally overlooks the many things that matter in between.

3) Sensitive dependence on initial conditions (SDIC)

The term, SDIC, tells us that it ain't always what you do or the way you do it. It's where and when you do it, that often makes the difference. And in complex systems, you can't always know for sure. Even the tiniest difference at the start, in any one of many parameters, can cause a significant difference in outcome somewhere down the line. SDIC is also known as the butterfly effect, where a butterfly flapping its wings, under precisely the right conditions, could in theory trigger a tornado. There is a big difference between knowing this, actually observing it, and finding a practical way to apply it.

Engineers create systems that deliberately amplify the effects of small things in predictable ways, so that, for example, a 70-year-old pilot can steer a jet with one hand. In more organic situations where we have no control over the design, the effect of small things can be surprisingly unpredictable.

The trouble is, we like to kid ourselves. Pharmacology invokes a theory from chemistry called the law of mass action, so that, loosely speaking, the response to a drug is a function of the dose. It would be nice if that were true, but the best we really get is a set of probabilities: the drug will save some people but kill others, and the prescription might need adjusting for the individual. Their nice, neat curve of dose against response is no practical law at all. It works in a test tube only, where the entire arrangement is kept as linear as possible.

In the real world, well-meant actions can backfire. A piece of bad luck can turn out to be a lifesaver. Small differences can sometimes change everything, against incredible odds. We see these effects all the time, and we even say, "That's life!"

I've adapted an example from James Gleick's *Chaos—making a new science* [1], the book that inspired me to take up physical sciences at university. Being unable to find your keys in the morning might normally be no big deal. You usually have a short wait for your train, so there is some tolerance in the plan. But suppose on one occasion, the phone rings and you talk for a minute. Then you spend another minute looking for your keys and get to the station moments too late to board the train. The next train is two hours later, and it's the slow train. So now you miss a morning at work because of a minute looking for your keys. And it happens also to be the morning where you had to give a vital presentation, to sell an idea to improve aircraft safety. Somebody else stands in for you, but they fluff the presentation. So, the company uses somebody else's product and, ten years later, a plane flies into the ground.

The way we see it, the crash has nothing to do with the keys, so a made-up example like this can seem far-fetched. But physics doesn't overlook a single thing. Similarly rare chains of events, good and bad, do happen quite literally all the time. It's just that there are too many interactions for us to see, and so we assign probabilities, happenstance, or divine intervention to explain events. Naturally, we try to contain the model, and look for points of predictability within it where we can make a difference. The trouble is complex systems are not so obedient as we would like.

So, even though the keys are causal, there is no repeat-ability, for all practical purposes. To prevent the next plane crash, there is a useful zone somewhere in between the lost keys and the plane actually dropping from the sky, where we might have some influence on the overall stability of the situation.

4) Fractals (pictorial abstractions of mathematical rules, that appear the same or similar at many different levels of magnification)

The striking images we call fractals could be seen as representing the narrow zone of unpredictability between regions of relative predictability, that all life must negotiate constantly in order to exist—the thin layer between the freezing cold of outer space and the searing heat of the earth's core for instance.

Fractals exhibit some startling features. One is the infinite detail of the swirls and wiggles in the boundary between two zones. That means, if you zoom in on the boundary, you can't tell at first which side of it you will land. An infinitesimal deviation can completely flip the result, and not always as you might expect.

Then there is the way that the whole can be seen in any of the parts. Zoom in as far as you like, and the pattern looks more or less the same, yet there can be an infinite variation of the details.

Features seen within a fractal can look hauntingly like things found in nature. Trees, snail shells, weather charts, human anatomy, snowflakes, coastlines, rivers, lightning strikes, eddies in water, smoke—can all seem to appear by magic out of some very simple sets of rules. Some of them possess a deeply unsettling quality as well.

Fractals seem to tell us something about knowledge. When you explore an idea, you find other ideas within, and other ideas within those.

Other graphics from Chaos theories tell us something about stability in dynamic situations. We can see a mathematical sequence of numbers orbiting a certain point on a graph, or even several points. The path never repeats, exactly, but stays within certain limits with each orbit, as long as the situation is stable.

Unavoidably, we must embrace the behaviour of complex systems as vital to our success. Within the ideas of chaos theory, there are a few important things to note. The obvious one is the breakdown of predictability. Another is that you simply never know what the myriad possible pathways are to cause situations, or to avoid and reverse them. And then there is a sense that almost everything in life is governed by chaotic laws, and that we can never escape that. But within the turmoil are recognisable patterns that can clarify things for us, even when the actual detail is confusing.

The reality check this gives to the healer is that it is far easier to say what general conditions might produce a more stable or less stable situation than to predict the precise results of a precise input.

In clinical practice, the ideal way to go is the one that depends on the right degree of specificity—not too general, not too precise. There is a necessary degree of breadth and subjectivity to this, and when in doubt, to err on the general side is usually the better mistake to make. It all brings us back to trusting the body, because if one thing is clear, it's that we really have very little idea what it is doing.

Medicine tries to tackle complexity by knowing more and more about how the body works, and finding more and more ways to measure what is going on in the patient, and then coming up with more and more precise ways to intervene. The hope is that eventually they will know enough to control any situation short of death itself.

But chaos tells us they never can know enough, nor even come close. So, the next solution is to have more and more specialists, who know more and more about less and less. But there can never be enough specialists. So, the hospitals get bigger and bigger, and the budgets get higher and higher.

Logically, the computer age can only compound this problem. Hospitals will keep getting bigger the more we know, but disease will not decrease one jot in that way.

Artificial Intelligence has no hope of solving this conundrum, not just because it cannot possibly ever know enough about what is going on inside the patient, even by taking them apart completely, but worse, because the people who design AI have got it looking in all the wrong places to begin with. There is another problem with AI, namely that it seems to lack any kind of mental homoeostasis, meaning that its algorithms can drift off insistently towards one pole or another and then stay there. Once it has made up its 'mind' about something, it becomes like a sort of authority to its masters, who forget that the AI depends on them changing their own minds in order to progress. New directions of thought will be rejected, because they go against the authority of the AI, like peer review, only worse.

The problems AI produces in medicine will be dealt with by applying yet more of the same, and the rewards of that approach will be ever more thorough symptom management, and lots of it. The cost will be a lifetime of dependence on therapy, followed by a truly horrific breakdown towards the end. This is predicable simply by extrapolating the current direction of medicine, which Phillip Day calls "entrenched scientific error: following the wrong course with the maximum of precision." [2]

With AI in medicine, the General Practitioner will become a thing of the past. You won't even have to wait until you feel sick. Your phone will go ping one day, you'll look and there will be the diagnosis of what the system thinks you are about to get. And there will be the QR code for the prescription. It will pester you to get it filled, and to take the drugs. And, who knows, if you don't, maybe public health will be called to check up on you, to protect the public, of course.

Scientists have gone so far as to try repairing our DNA, as if it has faulty bits that might simply be fixed.

This has got nowhere at all, not just because of the humungous technical obstacles, but because, frankly, they have very little idea about the true nature of what they are dealing with. Except in a tiny minority of examples, the faulty DNA hypothesis has proved to be a dud, as have all attempted solutions so far. Furthermore, variation is the basis of species success and the very engine of evolution: collectivists and atheists alike ought to *love* genetic variation. The notion of the 'defect' is a recent and inherently value-laden concept.

And so, the only possible routes to lasting systemic recovery are through natural laws and gross physiology.

In short, we need smarter ways to deal with complex systems, and throwing more and more computations at the problem isn't the answer. What we are looking for is not ways to catch falling cyclists and aeroplanes, but ways to bring our subject well within the limits where they can find their own easy stability once more and maintain it, and then step back and allow the wobbles to play out.

There is good news though. My belief is that we already had smarter ways—much smarter—it's just that they got shelved when chemical engineers took over medicine in the 20th century. And until they did, patients were generally on board. It does get even better, because when one drops the urge for technical micromanagement of cells and organs, all sorts of other ways to improve life suddenly become very accessible. The patient's problem is usually not a case of one huge weight on the camel's back. It is usually millions of straws. Precisely where the camel's back is breaking, and precisely which straw is responsible don't matter much when it comes to lightening the load.

Wernham's approach was to lighten the overall load by reducing stress in the posture, which had the bonus effect of simultaneously dealing with the lesion specifics indirectly, for all the reasons I have tried to explain. Had he chosen to work on specific adjustment instead of general treatment, the best he could have shown would be how to exchange one form of stress for another, with all the negative effects one would expect from that approach.

Even today, doctors and practitioners are looking for *the* single cause of every disease, or *the* specific cure. Likewise, many osteopaths believe in the key lesion, the one single thing in the body around which the entire disease state revolves. In chiropractic there are even those who specialise in adjusting a single bone—the atlas—believing that a disturbance there has to be the cause of all disease. They get great results, so they say. They also freely admit this approach includes recognising those who won't get better that way and discharging them. They call that ethical best practice. I call it cherry-picking.

The civil engineer builds an incredible bridge across the widest river and thus enables people to live where they might otherwise not choose to live. Defeating nature is the engineer's very purpose. In contrast, the artist or philosopher considers carefully where to live, and marries his home as best he can to his natural surroundings.

The engineer in medicine zooms in closer and closer on the cell, until he finds some misbehaviour in a protein to account for the patient's symptom. He offers to fix it, no context required. He builds a university. He gets paid well. He uses the power of the computer, the chemistry lab and the microscope to get as close as he can and makes an impressively precise correction. He defeats the body with the aim of curing it. Instead, it makes matters more complicated. So he applies for more funding. The philosophical healer zooms out. He walks a few easy steps back away from the symptom and wonders if partial dehydration could account for those same changes in the cells. He gives the patient a glass of water.

The key lesion is a myth. So is the uniquely consistent cause for every disease. They look for it, but they can't find it, except in the most proximate sense: the airway constriction was caused by asthma. Or else asthma is caused by airway constriction. I no longer know which it is supposed to be. But what is asthma? Oh, it's an autoimmune problem, they might say, which is another medical word for no idea, but let's start another medical school.

On the other hand, the further back you go looking for the cause, the more diffuse the trail becomes and the harder it is to find one single thing that really accounts for the problem. Could it be the keys? The phone call? Something else? But somewhere in between the two is a useful zone where you see many sets of interacting circumstances, with many more opportunities to help the system return to stability. This is the essence of indirect or non-linear treatment.

[1] James Gleick, book, *Chaos—making a new science*.

[2] Phillip Day, video, *Affairs of the Heart*, https://www.dailymotion.com/video/xe1hd9.

Missing Link 8: Fever and healing crisis

You don't need treatment. The fever, inflammation, coughing, etc., constitute the healing process. Just get out of their way and permit them to complete their work. Don't try to 'aid' nature. She doesn't need your puny aid—she only asks that you cease interfering.

—Herbert M. Shelton

The first time I left my osteopath's office and went into a high fever, I had no idea what it meant. I just assumed I had 'caught something' and went straight home to bed. I stayed there for two days, mainly just daydreaming, and as long as I just gave in to it and let myself rest, I felt okay. My parents had taught me how to manage a fever, and also not to see it as a big deal or anything to worry about. When I emerged, all my earlier aches and pains had gone and after another day or two, I felt positively energised. I was back at full throttle within the week.

What was really going on there I didn't know, and there was nobody to tell me. My osteopath at the time hadn't mentioned anything about it. A couple of years later, my wife had an intense fever that lasted almost a month, right after seeing a homoeopath. I called the homoeopath, and she said it was probably a *healing crisis*. I asked her if we should see a doctor and, I guess out of an abundance of caution, she said, "Maybe." I drove my wife to the hospital, where they took a quick look and said, "She's got a fever. So what? Take her home." They didn't think fever was cause for a freak-out. So, she spent the rest of that month resting in bed, waiting to come out of it. That was a turning point for things that had caused her trouble for years, and the beginning of the road to complete resolution.

I visited the same homoeopath and got a rash on my ankle, which disappeared in about a month. No apparent rhyme or reason to it, but, importantly, no problem either. But now that I had heard about something called the healing crisis, I was intrigued. During my training, I heard about it again, but only in passing. It was rumoured to be an illness that people can get on the way to recovery. But we had no systematic training in it, we weren't encouraged to bring such ideas into the clinic, or to try to invoke their potential; and definitely not to dabble in treating what was regarded as 'systemic illness'. It was only after college that I really tried to look into it, and found people who actually got its significance, and moreover employed it as an important weapon in their armoury.

The healing crisis can take the form of almost any acute symptom you can think of. The word 'crisis' doesn't mean emergency. It comes from an ancient Greek word for 'turning point in disease', and the word 'healing' qualifies it as positive.

Since becoming aware of it, I have noticed countless patients raise some kind of acute symptom picture following treatment, usually mild, that normally passes in a few hours to a couple of weeks and leaves them in better general condition. So many new patients have cancelled their follow-up appointments 'because of flu' that I can't count them.

Soon after graduating, I helped a young lady who had a new diagnosis of Multiple Sclerosis. Her symptoms were mild, and she was not yet at the stage of taking medication. Pretty soon she developed a head cold that lasted nearly two months and said that the most difficult thing about it was all the friends thrusting over-the-counter drugs at her and urging her to take them. When it went away, the tingles in her hands had gone and she remained largely free of symptoms for the next ten years or so. The last I heard about it, she was still living life to the full. Another case of misdiagnosis or spontaneous recovery?

So, what is going on? This goes back to the idea of the chronic resolving through the acute. The actual state of disease is often invisible: we see it most clearly through our body's attempts to recover. The acute symptoms invoked are healing processes, not disease. If you don't believe me, ask anybody you know with a lifelong chronic condition how often they get colds and flu. Never, hardly ever, or not for years, are the usual replies.

I have met people who have lost organs through cancer surgery yet tell me they are really healthy because they never get a cold. I have seen others raise their first cold in years, then immediately hit it with decongestants and painkillers. It is very difficult to offer them much when there is such a gulf between worldviews, and this may be one of the reasons our college advised us to generally avoid those cases. But cancer sufferers are not the only ones who may have learned an inverted view of health. Far from it. And to offer society much more than light pampering and mild pain-relief, some education is going to be needed.

Incidentally, I don't treat cancer. But there are people who come to me about other things, for whom cancer is a part of the overall picture.

The symptoms of a healing crisis can be almost anything but will often appear as something coming out of one of the various exit channels—the nose, the bowels, the lungs, the bladder—or onto the skin—boils, rashes, scabs, waxy substances, body odour, and so on. These are things on their way out of the body, as it works harder than usual to remove waste.

Following Hering's Law (mentioned earlier), aches and pains may appear as the focus descends from higher structures and functions to lower ones or moves from deep to superficial. Fevers are common. Fever is a more general healing process that renews and regenerates cells all over the body, destroys old and diseased ones, and increases immune system activity. Fever is often the first stage, and then more tangible discharges can follow later. But there is every permutation, and these things can go in any order.

I did see one man for neck pain, and his initial healing crisis consisted of diarrhoea and fever. Then, an old troublesome tooth went rotten and, without my prompting, he went and had it extracted. After that, his eardrum ruptured and some kind of discharge flowed out. Once all that was out of the way, his previously high blood pressure had come right down, and last of all, his neck pain finally went away. Clearly neither of us expected any of that to happen, not from a light treatment for a sore neck. It wasn't a load of fun for him, but he was delighted with the end result.

Importantly, someone less cool about matters would likely have had the process crushed medically at any of those stages, and then we would never have seen the natural outcome. I asked a colleague why the body would sacrifice its own eardrum if the point was to preserve bodily integrity. He replied, "Perhaps it spared him from meningitis or something. You'll never know."

Although there is no accepted modern biomedical theory to explain how a general spinal tune-up could have caused all that, by the same token, there is plenty of deniability for the practitioner. And I believe most practitioners would rest on that. Many of my colleagues would claim never to see healing crises, and some assert they are a myth. My guess is they see them all the time, and don't think to associate them with their work. What they infer is incidental illness, but more often they aren't even made aware of it, since the patient usually doesn't think to tell them.

But whether or not we think it important, or helpful, or safe, I don't think we can avoid it, since the body will exhibit these processes with or without our help. What matters is how they are managed and, they are only loosely related to our therapies. There is no way to plan them, or predict them, but we may sometimes have a clue that they are brewing. In that sense, we can't stop them either; not safely. Our therapy might make it easier or more likely for the body to start it, but the body will start it anyway, when it needs to and providing it gets the chance. Changes of season, a holiday, a new job, and more, can all kick off something. I'm sure we've all had a trip somewhere 'ruined' by sickness, and probably blamed it on a local restaurant, or a chap with a runny nose next to us on the plane (who is probably blaming us). It's not ruined: recovery is what a holiday is for.

Changes in lifestyle, habits and environment, especially good changes, can all set up favourable conditions for a bit of spring cleaning by the body: like the cough a smoker gets for a few weeks after quitting. Healing crises can often go around whole families, all around the same time. There are a number of possible reasons for this, and contagion is actually quite far from the only plausible theory. For one thing, families and communities live under the same weather. Their physiology is more or less the same and tuned into the same sets of clues. There is also a strong mental element to a healing crisis. You need to feel safe before the body will invest the energy for it, and one of the cues for that is seeing others doing the same thing. Typically, members of a household will take turns: perhaps children first, then one parent, then the other.

In essence, what the body is doing is taking advantage of a reduction in stress to devote energy to maintenance tasks. When we are very busy with survival, we put off vegetative processes of repair and elimination of waste. Our bodies can only do so much at once. We can't train for a marathon and repair damaged cartilage in our joints fully at the same time.

Stressed people tend to develop habits that keep their adrenal and sympathetic nervous systems raised all the time, because once the tone comes down from high alert, they feel achy, tired, nauseous, worried even. They may experience joint pain, headaches, and much more, as precursors to a more obvious healing event. Money worries and other concerns may start nagging at them. Sensing all this, they may then go to the gym—self medicating with adrenaline, essentially—or lean on stimulants and distractions to avoid the 'comedown'. Or they may simply decide to work harder at solving their problems, when working easier might be better. Their holiday involves trekking rather than taking it easy on a beach. And the longer the comedown is put off, the more it is needed, until the flood can't be contained anymore. Then all it takes is one early night or some other relief from the chores of life, and suddenly they are in bed with the flu. If their habit then is to take paracetamol and get back to work too soon, then the process isn't complete, and their problems will become more deeply entrenched. Their tissues will change to accommodate the increased storage requirements when elimination is suspended. And as generalised inflammation sets in over the years, many organs and tissues will lose efficiency, making them feel generally far less energetic, and chronically so. Continuation down this path of delayed or suppressed cleaning and healing, then locks one into a pattern that can get harder and harder to escape.

Hence, the route to chronic disease is often through suppression of mild symptoms one way or another, eventually on to harder suppression as more difficult symptoms appear. And the route to recovery is in changing all of these habits; not just the habits of the busy person keeping busy, but also their strategies for keeping going when their body is telling them to take a break, and how they manage the changes when they do occasionally stop.

Clearly then, any general therapy that is based around the reduction of stress and the improvement of lifestyle is, at the very least, going to promote these natural, normal healing events. It can't be stopped, not if one is going to be well. As far as my own personal post-treatment fevers are concerned—I have had many—the trigger is the removal of mechanical stress. There follows a consequent availability of additional energy for healing that had all previously been bound up in the posture. As for my wife's homoeopathic healing crisis, who knows? The mechanisms are there, but it's sometimes hard to map out the exact thing that changed.

The good news is that a healing crisis is safe. People's methods of managing it may not be, however.

The human body does not self-destruct by simply deciding to go wrong in some catastrophic way. The drive towards survival is relentless. But one is certainly more vulnerable to all kinds of external disturbance during times of repair and maintenance. The good old approaches to managing light illness always apply—rest in a safe and calm environment, don't get dehydrated, let somebody else know what is going on. Call in sick and don't go to work.

Additionally, if there is no appetite to eat, then eating is not necessary. The idea that a sick person must eat to keep up his strength is silly nonsense. It is far better to rest the digestive system when it is saying it doesn't want to work. There may be exceptions, such as pregnancy, eating disorders, cases of marked chronicity or low vitality. Modifying the diet and keeping it light may be the way to go. But generally speaking, forcing down food isn't a good idea. Prolonged fasting, however, does need additional guidance beyond what I can include here.

One of the worst ways to manage a healing crisis is to take random over-the-counter drugs for the symptoms. The, thankfully few, times I have heard of a healing crisis turning problematic have been when someone has done exactly that. Seeking advice first might have been wiser. There may be far better ways to get comfortable, or there may not be; and very occasionally the relief is simply in knowing that this is temporary. That said, the moment the patient thinks they have had enough is usually right before things turn the corner. For any practitioner involved, gauging this requires sufficient clinical knowledge, knowing your patient well enough, being respectful of their personal beliefs, and keeping a good track of events.

Once one understands that over-the-counter medications do not offer any health benefit, that the symptoms are temporary and the process helpful, and that, however bad the acute, the effect of suppression can be worse, then the discomfort of a healing crisis is generally much easier to bear. All that painkillers prove is that a sick person can take poisons and still recover.

People do sometimes ask how to tell if their symptoms are a healing crisis or an illness. Honestly, I think they are pretty much the same thing, framed differently; unless there are some previously known background considerations, or additional clues that something isn't right, or some new insult to the body is suspected. Severity alone doesn't always give the answer, although something very severe, very sudden, or outside the patient's previous experience can mean a real emergency. But regardless, the management of normal illness and the healing crisis is the same: obey the symptoms initially, and deal with underlying causes as and when you get a break to do so. Seek advice for anything you aren't sure about.

The supposition that common acute illnesses, such as seasonal flu, are inherently dangerous to a reasonably healthy person, is wrong. People don't die from flu so much as from its complications, and that can often be traced either to underlying health problems, or to the way the situation is managed. In the United States, the figures for death from the flu may have been greatly exaggerated by bundling them together with pneumonia [1]. I believe pneumonia arises when there is exhaustion or some significant prolonged stress. Everyone I know who has had pneumonia concurs. So rest, and don't wait until you collapse before taking a break!

It is possible that, when taking into account other confounding factors—such as frailty, pre-existing medical conditions, malnutrition, poor management, and medication—the risk of death coming exclusively from flu is pretty small. Flu is certainly not something I'm personally afraid of—in fact, I welcome its benefits [2] [3]. If

I don't have something vaguely flu-like every year or two, I start to wonder what's wrong.

Pre-existing or underlying medical problems are terms that merit discussion as well, some other time, from how the situations arise to the medications involved. However, non-medical practitioners need to think carefully before taking on a case in the middle of a crisis, or where the person is very frail or under extensive medical management already. Not least, there are so many other inputs present beyond the practitioner's control or even awareness. When a chronic situation has been managed medically for years, the opportunity for a true change of direction can, unfortunately, be long gone.

As to hospital management of flu and other such problems, I have seen and heard of such nonsense approaches over the years that it's no surprise that some don't benefit from the care. Take, for instance, the lady I met with ankles six inches wide from oedema (fluid retention), who had been admitted with complications of flu. How it all started is a story in itself, and in my view, this was one of those medical quagmires that was completely avoidable. But anyway, for the first two and a half days, the staff refused her all water, until her husband demanded she be allowed some fluid. At that point, she was given some soup and started to get better. How things turned out for her in the end, I do not know.

I once had to stand by my mother around the clock, fending off one particularly determined nurse bringing paracetamol for a fairly high temperature. Urging her to check her own guidelines made no difference: the idea of not medicating was completely intolerable to her. It was only when I insisted she fetch a doctor that she backed off. The doctor agreed there was nothing to worry about, and paracetamol wasn't indicated.

What I can see is that whether or not bad management in hospital is really what causes a person to die, you can be pretty sure that it won't be 'medical treatment' written on the death certificate.

The point here is that the symptoms of flu are not themselves the threat, but a survival mechanism. When we defeat our survival mechanisms, we defeat ourselves. If there is anything seriously wrong—and there can be— *it is not the symptoms*. And the cure for the common cold is a red herring, because, quite simply, *the cold is the cure*.

In support of this position, during the Spanish Flu of 1918, the osteopathic hospitals in the United States recorded a death rate of 0.25%, while the medical hospitals experienced a massively higher death rate of between 30% and 68% [4]. This has been cited as evidence of the excellence of osteopathic care. Just as likely, they simply weren't killing their patients. The *medical* treatment recommended just before the October death spike was aspirin, and patients were given insane doses of up to 31.2g per day [5]. The possibility that many of the deaths were iatrogenic—caused by medical treatment—seems too obvious to overlook, but under the carpet it seems to have been swept.

Unravelling what really went on in the Spanish Flu could take a book in itself. Suffice to say it is possible that this dark episode was the most colossal medical screw-up of the 20th century. Painting it all as enemy action from microbes meant the mistakes were bound to be repeated sooner or later. We have seen the same cycles several times since, of overreaction—overtreatment—increased deaths—etc., including SARS in 2003 and Swine Flu in 2009. It all adds to the perception of a deadly pandemic and trains our minds for the next one.

It is therefore hard not to mention COVID, although the subject provokes so much division that I told myself I wouldn't go there.

Throughout 2020 and 2021, many of my colleagues feared that a patient would bring a cold into their clinics. My fear was that a patient having a normal healing crisis would bring the authorities into the clinic to quarantine us. Interestingly, no colleague I know, anywhere in the world, has *ever* had their business remotely implicated in any kind of outbreak, despite the close personal proximity involved in the work. Yet at no point did anyone from public health ask us for our views on staying safe and keeping well.

Whatever people think we have all recently been through, I don't think it needs a deadly disease to explain it. Every feature of that entire miserable episode can be explained some other way. This is hard for some to accept, especially those who had a relative in hospital at some point. But were it not for the unprecedented restrictions and non-stop fear-based messaging, who would have even thought there was something big happening?

To create a global health crisis, all one needs to do is to spread word of a deadly disease and let human nature do the rest. Why public health might shout "fire" in a crowded theatre is another discussion, but there is no doubt in my mind this is what we have just witnessed.

Pandemics are something that have intrigued me since college. And I dealt with 2020 through a prior framework of understanding, that pandemics are usually, if not always, things medicine calls pseudo-epidemics—self-fulfilling prophecies, essentially, where fear of disease causes more destruction than disease itself. In some cases people die from the panic measures, or from something entirely normal: they get recorded as victims of whatever is supposed to be circulating, and then the whole thing gathers momentum. Once the mistakes become apparent, officials and experts go into self-preservation mode, and then the truth gets garbled. The newspapers change the subject and it goes away. And here we are.

There is a real point to discussing pandemics here: they aren't exceptions to the theory of natural healing. They tell us nothing useful about disease, and everything about what can go wrong when superstition takes over. Paradoxically, they provide a very good reason *not* to get overexcited about common everyday symptoms.

By discussing what may actually be going on when we get ill—whether we call it illness or call it a healing crisis—hopefully this will help people to join a few dots, and most of all, not to panic about common illness. We will go deeper into this in the next chapter. I am not saying all the answers are known, but until this side of the conversation can be had in the open, they never will be.

Our grandparents didn't think every sniffle needed a drug. Nor did they think they needed antibiotics for every boil.

But even in my lifetime, I have noticed a huge loss of common knowledge in how to manage common everyday things that happen to all of us and that people used to take in their stride. This knowledge has been replaced by a fear of illness, fever especially. It is all geared towards medicalising everyday problems and turning our default setting to 'seek medical help'. And unless practitioners reclaim and redefine the meaning and progression of symptoms, they are depriving themselves of some of the sharpest tools in the box.

At this point, people often ask: "Can't a fever cause brain damage or convulsions?" The short answer is no, with the caveat that fever *can be associated with* serious outcomes, and it can also depend on how the symptoms are managed. For example, you can die from malaria, say, but it is not the fever which kills you. The fever is trying to save you. If medical treatment is needed, it is for the underlying problem; in this case, generally thought to be a blood parasite.

More importantly, lowering a fever does nothing to improve the outcome, except perhaps to make the patient more comfortable. In fact, UK medical guidelines say as much, a point I have had to argue hot with hospital staff more than once. Antipyretic (fever-lowering) drugs can be highly detrimental.

Dr Robert Mendelsohn's excellent little book, *How to raise a healthy child in spite of your doctor*, goes into this in much more detail [6]. He points out that febrile convulsions in children—the fear parents often raise—precede the fever and are to do with how quickly the fever rises, not how high it goes. In other words, if you know the child has a fever, convulsions would have already happened, if they were going to. Giving fever-lowering drugs therefore does not prevent convulsions. Why they happen is, of course, another matter. Suffice to say they are not normal or common, and prompt medical advice should be sought.

None of this is to advise against seeking medical help for someone with a fever if you are worried, especially a baby. Fever in a baby is not normal either. The point is to view things from another perspective: to look beyond the fever, recognise what it may signify, and deal with that if necessary. Then we might feel more confident about managing things at home, but also recognise more swiftly when medical intervention is in fact needed.

Mendelsohn goes on to explain that the temperature of a fever alone, even a high one, bears no relationship to the seriousness of the problem. And the temperature can't just keep on rising and rising to a dangerous level, since fever is a regulated and necessary physiological process. The heat comes from the metabolic activity of cells, and there is an upper limit to their output, just as there is an upper limit to how fast a car can go.

I don't wish to address specific fever management here. There are many works on that already, and I would support the ones that emphasise not trying to bring down the temperature simply because it is up.

In spite of the huge amount of fear and suspicion surrounding fever, its power to overcome disease has long been known about. One of the most effective cancer cures ever developed was when Dr William Coley found ways to provoke fever [7]. He noticed that those who developed high temperatures after cancer surgery were far more likely to recover.

I am not saying that Dr Coley's methods were without flaws: there is a big difference between a spontaneous healing event and a deliberate purge. A purge stresses the body to provoke an intended reaction, whether it wants it or not. In contrast, a healing crisis is something the body chooses to do, after it has been relieved of stress. The two are not the same.

The fear of fever arises partly from superstitions that abound in society, and partly from the fact that serious illness can be associated with fevers. But it is arguably part of the psychology of the great medical land grab. While it is perhaps understandable that some people fear fever, it is not logical to try and stop it as a matter of routine. Yet, if someone happens to be lucky enough to raise a fever while in hospital, staff will often come along armed with paracetamol, saying, "That's all you need on top of everything else!" It is probably exactly what they do need.

[1] Doshi P. *Are US flu death figures more PR than science?* BMJ 2005; 331 :1412 doi:10.1136/bmj.331.7529.1412.

[2] Herbert Shelton, *The Rationale of Fever,* The Hygienic System, Volume IV—Orthopathy, Chapter III.

[3] Erika Duffell, *Curative power of fever,* The lancet, Volume 358, ISSUE 9289, P1276, October 13, 2001

[4] Harold I. Magoun, Jr, D.O., *More About the Use of OMT (Osteopathic Manipulative Treatment) During Influenza Epidemics,* Journal of the American Osteopathic Association, Oct 2004.

[5] Karen M. Starko 2009, *Salicylates and Pandemic Influenza Mortality,* 1918–1919 Pharmacology, Pathology, and Historic Evidence, Clinical Infectious Diseases, Volume 49, Issue 9, 15 November 2009, pp. 1405–1410.

[6] Dr Robert Mendelsohn, book, *How to raise a healthy child in spite of your doctor*.

[7] Stephanie Pain, *Dr Coley's Famous Fever*, New Scientist, 2 Nov 2002, https://www.newscientist.com/article/mg17623675-700-dr-coleys-famous-fever/.

Missing Link 9:
Terrain Theory

If I could live my life over again, I would devote it to proving that germs seek their natural habitat—diseased tissue—rather than being the cause of dead tissue. In other words, mosquitoes seek the stagnant water, but do not cause the pool to become stagnant.

—Dr Rudolph Virchow

Two important ideas have competed for centuries:

1) Germ Theory loosely says that exposure to micro-organisms is the cause of infection and disease.

2) Terrain Theory, many would say, is that germs merely exploit the unhealthy, that microbes are the product of disease, not the cause. They are like the flies around the dung-heap, but they didn't produce the dung, so to speak.

So, which is right? A bit of both, maybe? And why does it matter?

The important point is that microbes need a suitable habitat (terrain) in which to live, so if you want to stay healthy, fighting germs will only get you so far. It is up to you to have to maintain your inner health.

Taking an ecological view, it seems perfectly reasonable that we would have developed some kind of harmony with our little friends sharing planet earth with us. If we regularly ride on London Transport, we are surely exposed to just about every pathogen known, yet we aren't all dead. It certainly isn't the biggest challenge to most Londoners' health. From this common-sense perspective, terrain theory is a clear winner already. But it goes much deeper than that, and the ramifications are huge.

Antoine Béchamp was Louis Pasteur's lesser-known contemporary, who really brought the study of microbes into the scientific age. Béchamp, who was without doubt the better scientist, tried to understand the place of germs in the ecology of humans, while Pasteur, the better social climber, levered his connections to declare war on them; a war we have been fighting, at great cost, ever since.

Pasteur was well aware of Béchamp's work: he took the bits he liked, rejected the bits he didn't like, and monetised the most simplistic interpretation. He developed dubious and even dangerous biologics, on the promise of ridding the world of disease by saving us from germs. He spun his results to claim effectiveness whenever there was none. The fact that he gained so much attention for his research and products has perhaps more to do with his social connections than the true value as therapeutics. What he proposed were bolt-on solutions that required no real attention to the environmental causes of disease. It is easy to see why that was a very attractive proposition to backers, politicians and the public—if only it might have worked.

Béchamp offers more than a different viewpoint. He actually turns germ theory completely inside out. I would urge anyone who is interested to read Ethel Hume's, *Béchamp or Pasteur: a lost chapter in the history of biology* [1]. This explosive history is essential reading for any natural therapist; and, I suggest, for any doctor serious about purging medicine of its limiting superstitions.

The first challenge of Terrain Theory is to the idea of self and separateness. Germs do not just live in us, but they are part of us at a physiological level. We are an ecology that inhabits, more or less, the outlines of our bodies, and exists within a much larger global ecology. The division between us and everything else is very blurry indeed. Our tissues can become 'not us'. You only have to get athlete's foot to know this is true.

Today, microbiology even recognises endogenous viruses that come from our own DNA; the prevailing theory being that they planted their coding there as an adaptive ploy. But if we forget man-made ideas like self and non-self, then all we can really say is that most bacteria and viruses found within us are mere features of our own physiology.

Béchamp pre-dates the modern theory of viruses, but the virus is something we need to mention in this context. As covered in an earlier chapter, there are surprisingly few hard facts about viruses. However rigorous and detailed modern virology and its various spin-offs seem to be, they cannot be relied upon, since they, in turn, depend on inferences and deductions, from beliefs that lack a truly solid foundation. Few people would believe how much superstition, unfounded assumption, circular reasoning, guesswork, and frankly atrocious science are involved when a virus is identified and characterised.

I suggest reading Janine Roberts' superb, *Fear of the Invisible* [2], to get a sense of just how shockingly pseudoscientific virology actually is. What we call viruses may be little more than cellular debris, or at most, the output of failing cells that need replacing (exosomes). The means to identify them are cranky, to say the least, and the conclusions formed about what they are and what they are supposed to do lack any sound logic. In the modern age, computer programmes, rather than actual laboratory findings, fill many of the gaps in the knowledge.

But when talking about microbiology in general, the broad point remains that there is not an outside and inside world; it is certainly impossible to say where one ends and the other begins.

Another special case, not known about until quite recently, is Prion Disease, such as Mad Cow Disease (Bovine Spongiform Encephalopathy, BSE). This is a conundrum that has really only appeared on a worrying scale following some pretty unnatural practices. The supposed pathological process in sheep scrapie, BSE, and Kuru in Papua New Guinea, doesn't need too much detail for this argument. The point is that the official version has some very good rival theories.

The theory that Kuru is caused by cannibalism, is based on anthropological myths and the unreliable testimony of a few explorers [3].

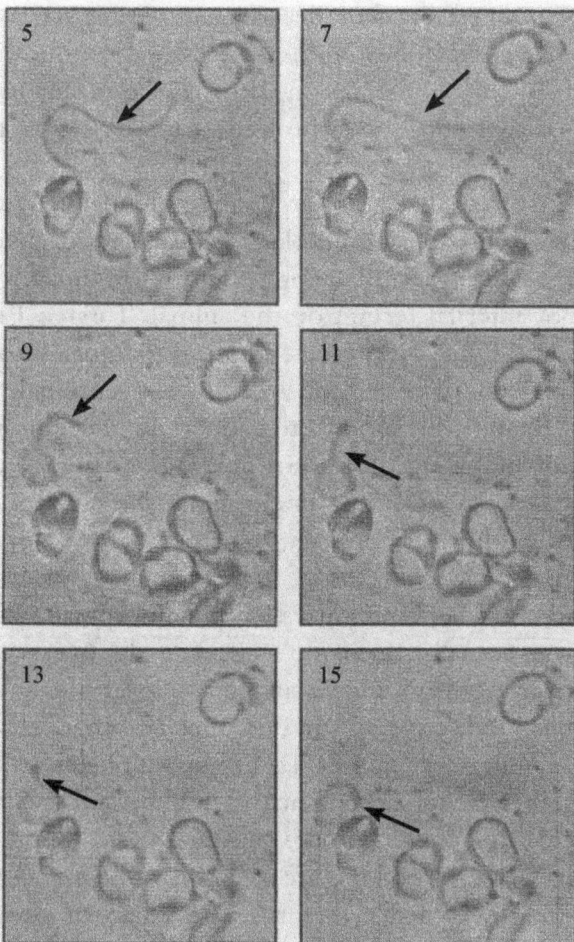

Pleiomorphic change in a live blood sample, caught on camera.
A rod-type bacterium transforms into a spherical cell, like a coccus
bacterium or one of the adjacent blood cells. In conventional biology this isn't thought possible. From *Sick and Tired, reclaim your inner
terrain*, by Dr Robert Young, PhD, DSc and Shelley Young, LMT.
Reproduced with permission.

BSE is an effect of modern farming. Some say copper deficiency is the culprit. Others say that BSE follows the use of Warble Fly spray on cattle. Since pesticides are neurotoxic, it's a good hypothesis. One has to wonder, therefore, about scrapie and sheep dip.

The truth is that there are many potential candidates for the causes of the neurological degeneration blamed on prions, and they all accord one way or another with the poor internal terrain of the animal. Torsten Engelbrecht and Claus Köhnlein's, *Virus Mania* goes into this in some detail [3]. Even the accepted conventional prion disease theory still amounts to bad terrain; the tainting of the body by eating things not normally in the diet. But its fundamental scientific underpinnings seem to be no better than those of virology.

Further down the rabbit hole than most of us will venture is a phenomenon called pleiomorphism [1] [4]. This was actually Béchamp's startling discovery about what really goes on in cells and sub-cellular life, and has since been rediscovered and described by other researchers in one form or another. Talking about pleiomorphism is not a recipe for acceptance in science and medicine. But here goes. Bacteria, fungi, and countless other microorganisms are part of the life cycles of our own cells and their sub-components. In turn, we are part of their life cycle that happens to be in a gross (large scale) colonial phase.

Putting it another way, human cells, bacteria, and fungi are the same stuff, made of the same smaller elements, just doing different things under different conditions. And crucially, what Béchamp realised is that they can turn into each other and back again as conditions change. The components of a cell can reorganise to make a bacterium. This flies completely against accepted modern biology, which says that one thing can only consume another, it cannot change directly into it. There are many possible objections to pleiomorphism, but none are fatal. The definitive answers ought to be found in evidence, and that means research. Good luck getting funding to study human cells turning into bacteria and back again, though. To the scientific establishment, this is as heretical as turning lead into gold. Not least, it threatens the idea that there is a blueprint for life contained entirely in our DNA, and the fortunes that ride on that theory. But imagine what doors might be opened if there were more to it?

I guess that any microbiologists reading this will disagree strongly with some of the points. But if they can take on board the essence of the argument and pursue it, they may still discover better truths than the ones they already have.

And so, the second challenge is to the cell as the basic unit of life. Even a school child can see that the cell can be divided into smaller elements, some of which even have their own DNA (e.g., mitochondria). Even by conventional biology, we see disorganisation and reorganisation take place as part of normal cell activity. So why exactly we are told cells are the basic building blocks of life is itself a mystery; perhaps to obfuscate the reality?

But then it gets quite strange. The sub-units of cells are themselves divisible smaller and smaller. Many levels of division beneath the cell have been observed. That's a whole universe that modern microbiology doesn't mention. The smallest unit, according to Béchamp, is the microzyme, and microzyma (plural) not only appear to be indivisible as life forms but are incredibly enduring. Béchamp showed that chalk from ancient rock beds could initiate fermentation in a sugar solution, just as if it contained living yeast. This same was not achieved using sterile calcium carbonate made in the lab. Critics say he must have been sloppy, but his experiments were rigorous. It seems as if microzyma contain enough information somehow to at least kick-start the organisation of simple organic molecules into primitive life-forms, and to direct the process.

The organisation of microzyma into cells remains while higher life persists. The microzyma support the higher structure until cell death (disorganisation), after which they then become 'liberated' and reorganise themselves as the building blocks for a new kind of organisation. They don't commit suicide just because we die. They march happily onwards to the next phase of their life cycle, becoming bacteria, fungi, and so on.

You don't need a special microscope to see this in action: just try cutting open an over-ripe avocado. You will see rings of decay, taking place as a reorganisation from within, not consumption from without.

Béchamp observed cacti that had been frozen in cold weather and found bacteria deep within them where nothing could have penetrated from outside. The frozen tissue is not dead, it is just disorganised, and when it thaws, it automatically begins reorganising itself. He performed rigorous lab versions that showed the same phenomenon.

And were you to cut open a corpse, you would find nothing dead inside it; just life reorganising itself from one state into another. Corporeal death is therefore little more than a switch from one level of organisation to another.

Some of this strange Béchampian behaviour can be seen on a larger scale. Slime-moulds are organisms appearing as little more than an amorphous soup with no dividing membranes, yet they behave as if highly organised, highly coordinated, and even with what appears to be some level of intelligence [5]. They can at times exhibit higher structural organisation, complete with fruiting bodies like fungi, and then lose it again.

The implications for health are not trivial. When our tissues become diseased, the components of the cells act as if we are dead and switch into the next phase of their life cycle, becoming bacteria, yeast, and so on.

That athlete's foot is a clue to where this is going on. One of the body's ways of dealing with acidic waste is to push it onto the skin. The overgrowth between the toes is a local sign of this mechanism working hard: bacteria and fungi thrive in acidic environments. The tissues there lose their support, and reorganisation begins. The fungus may even be keeping us alive by drawing out waste. You can't spread the fungus to other toe spaces—I've tried. But nor can you fix the problem with fungicidal ointment, since it always comes back.

So, significantly, bacteria and fungi are not creators of the disease state, but *the result* of the disease state. Kill the bacterium and the disease remains, to re-emerge later in some other form. This explains why the futile war on

germs, started by Pasteur, Lister, and others, has failed to
solve the problem of disease overall.

The problem is not so much the bacterium, which
can usually pass in and out of our bodies unnoticed.
The problem is the dead and putrid matter that typically
comes along as part of the package. You could culture
the bacteria from faeces and consume them in their pure
state without any harm. These days they call it a probiotic
and sell it. It is the solid morbid matter in the faeces that
causes the most harm when it enters the body, particularly through an open wound.

Béchamp and others showed that bacteria and fungi
are involved in reorganising the breakdown products of
disorganised tissue into a new state. If this seems confusing, bear with me.

The thinking goes that, out of our own tissues, our
bodies can produce the very precise bugs we need to
clean up waste, package it all up, contain it safely, and
help transport it out of the body. Dr Robert Young calls
this 'outfection' [4]. It is the toxins within diseased tissues
that are the real issue, and the regulation and support to
those tissues … not the germs. If the microbial link in
the chain of elimination is taken away, then this pathway
is thwarted. The toxins must be addressed by the rest of
the system, some other way, and the general disease state
remains or even deepens.

Antibiotics may be one way to improve the appearance of diseased tissues; not simply because they kill bacteria, but because in doing so, they force the body to stop
putting out waste through that route. They then load up
the patient in some other way.

When the germs themselves die this way, they break apart and can dump their toxic load back into the body, in some cases causing a dangerous reaction called a Herxheimer Reaction. Misguided therapists will often mistake this for a healing crisis after using some other means, besides antibiotics, to target the bacterium directly. And this is why fixation on the microbe can be counterproductive even in so-called natural methods. It works counter to the body's natural processes for addressing disease, and calling the result a healing crisis shows an inadequacy of understanding.

The general idea of targeting cells—whether cancer cells, bacteria, single-celled parasites or whatever—as if causal agents, should at the very least be considered with caution. They are crude intentions based on a crude understanding. Rife machines, for instance, have gained renewed attention lately for their ability to 'zap' cells with specific frequencies. There is far less attention however, to Royal Rife's earlier discoveries about the terrain. Rife saw great importance in understanding why diseased cells and microbes appear in the first place through biological transformation. I doubt he intended his brilliant invention to be used as just another antibiotic, and I have known people get into trouble using Rife machines that way.

Far from being victims of bacteria, it seems we are farming them and culling them according to our needs. On the other hand, antibiotics upset the ecology between our own cells and those that live on us. In doing so, they block our own secretions that we depend upon to control the balance. Our secretions, capable of killing some of the worst of the so-called antibiotic-resistant strains, depend on signalling from our gut bacteria to our own cells: no normal gut bacteria, no signalling, no antiseptic secretions [6] [7]. Thus, hospital superbugs are, in effect, man-made organisms whose ideal niche is hospital patients on antibiotics.

The sterility of the hospital environment itself may be making matters worse. All that toxic hand sanitiser and scrubbing of door handles is utterly missing the point. It creates a microbial vacuum for nature to fill. It certainly doesn't seem to have solved the problem of hospital superbugs. This over-emphasis on germs instead of dirt is, in fact, adding to the dangers of being in hospital. The conventional view that bacteria become superbugs through breeding selection—the strong ones simply survive the antibiotics—is manifestly incomplete.

Hospitals are toxic places already, and over-sterility is, in fact, incompatible with life. Animals reared experimentally in completely aseptic conditions do not survive more than a few days—another interesting point from *Virus Mania* [4]. There is no way to keep them alive. Filling a patient's environment with various biocides can only add to their toxic burden, and smearing dirt around the place with disinfectant doesn't really help.

True enough, not all bacteria are our friends. It is also true that bacteria exhibit an unimaginable range of lifestyles, many of which we know nothing about. Indeed, once established in the body, some bacteria can maintain the conditions for their own proliferation, making it harder to overcome them. And there are, of course, bacteria that can poison us through their secretions. But most are of no consequence whatsoever, and many have a positive contribution to make.

Again, the issue with hostile bacteria is susceptibility: human health and inner terrain, in other words.

For example, Listeria requires rotting food such as milk in order to proliferate, and in most of us, it causes no problems anyway. Listeriosis is associated with lowered stomach secretions and the use of antacids. We have an ample warning system through well-functioning senses of smell and taste. Botulinum doesn't survive in oxygenated situations, and a healthy body with good circulation is well-oxygenated. People with normally functioning immune systems are not at risk from the bacterium itself. The toxin it produces, however, is very dangerous, and can travel into us in tainted food. Where it proliferates, producing lots of toxin, is in anaerobic environments, such as sealed tins of meat. This is a consideration for the packaging and processing industry.

The point here is that even harmful bacteria do not use our own healthy tissue as a substrate for growth; there has to be some compromise in the terrain, or the insertion of foreign matter for it to live on. Tetanus is mainly a problem of poor wound management: a well-washed wound free of dirt is the most effective prevention. The list is huge of potentially deadly bacteria that can quite commonly live in us at a low level while hardly causing our immune systems to blink. If they get out of hand, it is because something else has gone wrong in our terrain.

And if we don't understand how our therapy interacts with the patient's natural immunity, we risk either harming them, or missing powerful opportunities to heal.

And thus, our missing links start to join up.

One part of our terrain is to do with our toxic state (Missing Link 5). Another is tissue regulation via nerve and blood, and that is where structural adjustment fits in (Missing Link 6). When we get an illness, it is our body's way of 'cleaning house' (Missing Link 8), and we suppress that to our cost.

If, every time our patient has symptoms, they are hit too directly (Missing Link 7—Chaos and complex systems) with antipyretics, anti-inflammatories, or antibiotics, sooner or later those measures will stop working and he will be messed up (Missing Link 4—Progression of disease).

So, what can we do instead? With a coherent roadmap (Missing Link 2) to guide strategy, we can anticipate and avoid the negative effects of a reactive approach. We can see more clearly where the events of recovery are heading and think several moves ahead.

If we regard infection as something coming out instead of something trying to get in, then we can consider the areas of general stress and susceptibility—the toxic state, deficiencies, nutritional issues, disruption to normal regulation. We can offer remedies that help neutralise and draw out waste, or nutrients and fluids that are needed in excess at certain times. We can employ any number of means to keep the mechanisms of regulation in tune, and the pathways of elimination clear. And we can do all this without waiting for germs to show up, meaning we can also perhaps prevent a septic issue from arising in the first place.

And yes, it does help, sometimes when medical therapy has failed completely. This is why even fairly blunt vitamin C therapy can work so well, through offering useful antioxidant support. It isn't an antiviral or antibiotic in the direct sense, but it has the effect of making unwanted microbes disappear.

Or we can just leave things well alone, as long as the body seems to be on top. In other words, we can do less. Where and when we do act, we can do so with a different emphasis.

And we can see the germ, not as a specific enemy, but as one possible consequence of a more general state of depletion or enervation. Whatever intervention follows from that, at the very least, *it must not deplete or enervate the patient further.*

Perhaps it is now apparent why the lack of deeper philosophy makes modern medicine such a faux pas, and why medicine's involvement makes it so much harder for us to do anything useful for the health.

Using antibiotic and antimicrobial chemicals as a means of control is crude and harmful, since it destroys more or less indiscriminately, like throwing Agent Orange over a rainforest. When the forest eventually grows back, what appears is not the same as before. Once a new equilibrium is established, no amount of selective planting will restore the old balance. This is a main cause of gut dysbiosis, candida infestations, and worse, and it takes more than a few probiotic supplements to overcome it.

As to our immune systems, they are essentially our waste recognition and removal system. Much of innate immunity is pretty passive and is about keeping the doors closed to that which is harmful. The task of the rest is to identify anything non-self, dead or malfunctioning inside the body, render it harmless and get it out safely if it can. Gobbling up microbes is but a very specialised task within that. But our white cells, often poetically called soldier cells, ought really to be called bin-bag cells, because that is what they are—garbage containers—and anything more flowery is totally anthropomorphic.

In death, we see life continue on a smaller scale, but a loss of the organisation of the whole. We see new organisation arise from within the old. Life within us endures, even after what makes us 'us' has gone. In disease of the higher organism, gross coordination begins to break down, and the smaller units of life begin to reclaim their primacy. And thus, living nature endures and propagates. The smallest units of all are incredibly hardy, capable of persisting in desert, 60-million-year-old chalk, polar ice caps, and perhaps, on comets and asteroids.

What Béchamp destroys is the 'us and them' vision of health and disease, which is a construct of the human imagination. Yes, we have complex and varied relationships with microbes. Yes, there could be communication and transmission of systemic behaviour, which we might call contagion, but which we might also call something else. In many examples, contagion is an illusion anyway. Things come in clusters for all kinds of reasons, and attempts to solve viral contagion have consistently failed, once we look behind the facades of many supposed medical triumphs [8]. Is the cure for the common cold coming any time soon? As it turns out, we still don't know for sure how to spread one (Missing Link 5).

What Béchamp doesn't give us is something we can easily package and market. It leads to careful, painstaking solutions that won't make one rich and famous.

If further evidence were needed, it is that the huge reductions in infectious disease during the last two centuries have come from measures such as plumbing and food management. Great systems for keeping our bodily waste as far away as possible, and bringing fresh food and clean water into our cities, have done the most to keep us healthy.

As holistic practitioners then, our aim remains to promote healthy living, assist the systems of the body to remain organised and coordinated, and thereby keep the body clean on the inside. Once again, it all leads to low-tech solutions that are tolerant of error, and towards self-reliance and less centralised forms of healthcare.

[1] Ethel D Hume, book, *Béchamp or Pasteur: a lost chapter in the history of biology*.

[2] Janine Roberts, book, *Fear of the invisible*.

[3] Torsten Engelbrecht and Claus Köhnlein, book, *Virus Mania*.

[4] Robert O Young, Shelley Young, book, *Sick and Tired*.

[5] The Lowen Foundation, video, *Seifritz on Protoplasm - Full Film*, https://youtu.be/_ihSxAn4WR8.

[6] Ute Schönfelder, *Bacterial toxin with healing effect*, Friedrich-Schiller-Universitaet Jena, Science Daily 13 Oct 2020, https://www.sciencedaily.com/releases/2020/10/201013134304.htm.

[7] Piccioni A, Rosa F, Manca F, Pignataro G, Zanza C, Savioli G, Covino M, Ojetti V, Gasbarrini A, Franceschi F, Candelli M, *Gut Microbiota and Clostridium difficile: What We Know and the New Frontiers*. Int J Mol Sci. 2022 Nov 1;23(21):13323, doi: 10.3390/ijms232113323. PMID: 36362106; PMCID: PMC9657115.

[8] Suzanne Humphries and Roman Bystrianyk, book, *Dissolving Illusions*.

Missing Link 10: Vitality

*I never, ever, touch fried food ... And I never run
for a bus. There'll always be another.*

—Mel Brooks, 'The 2000 Year Old Man'

There is a theory that we are born with a certain allot-
ted number of heartbeats, and that when they have
all been used up, we die. Others talk about a finite number of breaths. The logical inference is that there is a balance to be met, between using them as slowly as possible,
and at the same time using them well enough to get things
done so we can feed ourselves, and to maintain adequate
physical condition. I'd say it is partly true.

Indeed, people whose lifestyles demand high cardiac
output don't always live long. Endurance athletes, and
those with intensely physical jobs, can and do acquire
chronic health problems. They may nevertheless soldier
on in spite of these problems, believing that an intense
exercise regime is the way to overcome them. It is easy to
overlook the importance of rest.

Stagnation is of course a killer too. But there is reason
to believe that we have got the association the wrong way
around—and that exercise is a marker of health, not a
cause of health. It's not that more exercise makes people
healthier, it's that healthier people exercise more because

they can. And generally speaking, injury and exhaustion are greater obstacles to fitness than the amount of training.

So, exercise is certainly connected with health: but there is only a slight overlap between health, beauty, and athletic performance. Physical tempering in youth can prepare us for life. But what keeps us healthy is *movement*. And if athletic gains are desired, intensity-based training is generally more useful than endurance training.

Long ago I read about activity in school children—I wish I could find the study. Apparently, those who are made to exercise more in the day, play less vigorously in the evening. And those without access to sport at school tend to run around more when they get home. In other words, children—and perhaps adults—naturally adjust their exercise to what is right for them. My extrapolation is that for an unhealthy person to force himself to the gym may not be such a good idea as it sounds.

There are plenty of reasons why such intensity may lead to a shortened life and ill health. For starters, the demands of relentless physical output cause great stress on all the organs, not just the joints and muscles.

Additionally, the athletic body makes adaptations that are aligned with short-term crisis survival, a bit like preparing for war. Less energy goes into vegetative processes needed for a long life, such as regeneration, assimilation of nutrients, repair of damage, considering one's place in the universe, and so on. Those other processes also require energy, and they mostly take place during periods of rest, reflection and recovery, when the muscles aren't using it all up. When an extended crisis is over and we take a break, that is often when we feel the pain. The aches return as the muscles recover. The joints may become inflamed as damaged cartilage repairs itself. Old physical symptoms and pains rise to the surface and the mental demons return. Over time, the weight goes on as we replace the resources we have used up, ready for the next crisis. This is assuming, of course, that our organs can still cope with the workload of digestion, and aren't too depleted, or packed with waste, to do the work.

The physical and mental comedown after an event, or the completion of a project, or a separation from a stressful partnership, can be huge. This is why people get colds and flu whilst on summer holidays. It is why families fight at Christmas. Ironically, it is also why people with arthritis are told to keep exercising, on the basis that the relief from inflammation signifies some kind of healing. More likely, it signifies the suppression of our primary repair process while the joints are doing work. Working a badly worn joint hard, makes no more sense than driving faster with a flat tyre.

I meet people who say they have to keep working because when they stop, their immune system collapses and they get sick. Nothing could be further from the truth. It is when they stop that their immune system finally has a chance to catch up on some unfinished business. And there may be a lot of unfinished business.

I meet habitual runners who have to run miles every day because otherwise they 'go crazy'. It's not that sitting still causes them mental problems, it's that running masks them. They are quite literally self-medicating with adrenaline. And there are those who can't get through their busy days without six cups of coffee.

The problem is that nobody can sustain this approach indefinitely. And if they try, they will be on a path that can lead to burnout, or infertility, or medication so they can digest their lunch safely, or some other effect of chronic stress and the adaptations to heavy workloads. At some point, if they don't slow down or stop, reality will force them to anyway, and not on pleasant terms.

Chronic problems such as adrenal fatigue do not normally happen to lazy people, and there is nothing that can replace actual rest and recovery. Offering 'adrenal support' can be misguided, and can help a driven person get further into the corner. Recovery can take years, during which they must be very gentle on themselves at all times, especially in the early stages. Otherwise, any little bit of slack they find can get gobbled up, catching up on all the things they have been waiting to sort out. In fact, most of us probably live somewhere in the zone between adequate regeneration and some kind of degenerative breakdown caused by our lifestyles. If at times we find ourselves struggling to keep going, it is best to heed the warnings, or else more severe warnings will follow.

And supporting a high output with super-nutrition might not be the way either; in much the same way that fitting high performance parts to an old engine may help it burn more fuel and go faster but does nothing to stop it wearing out. Particularly when one is consuming large amounts of vitamins and super-foods, they may tend to mask a problem that is fundamentally not about their lack, but about the demands on the body. It is possible that flooding the organs with complex nutrients, to compensate for the effects of stress and dysregulation, simply adds to the overall workload. It may be decades before we really know the full effect—beneficial or otherwise—of this approach.

So, I don't think this equation all boils down to a predetermined number of heartbeats or breaths, since there are far too many other variables. But when somebody came up with the idea of a lifetime limit to our aggregate output, they were onto something all the same. The flaw was in tying it all to a single crude variable.

The natural hygienists once recognised a more general concept called 'vitality' or 'vital energy'. Counting heartbeats is simplistic, whereas vitality is one of those simple ideas out of which arises a great deal of sophistication.

We are endowed with a finite amount of vital energy and use it up during our lives. It is not known where exactly this comes from, when it arrives, or what physical quantities it represents. But it is there, and once it is all gone, we die. There is no way to get it back. The exact amount we are blessed with cannot be measured, but it may, perhaps, be estimated, and it is different for everybody.

Some of us have a lot, and some of us have a little, and we can use it at different rates, depending on the demands on our systems at different times. So, it is possible for somebody with a huge amount of vitality to use it all up rapidly and die young, and it is also possible for somebody with much less to use it very sparingly and live much longer.

One should not judge a book by its cover, and in health no less so. A snapshot of a person showing the appearance of health may suggest great vital energy, but it could be a sign of it being burned through at a high rate, or their problems being internalised to a great extent. Nor does an outward appearance of poor health say much about the journey they are on. Many people have survived experiences that would have killed others, and the fact that they are still going at all is evidence of an incredible natural resilience. As practitioners, it is useful to try and gauge which it is. It may also be that somebody has high vitality, but they appear depleted and drained, because their output is being used inefficiently in some way, or being allocated to addressing a lifetime of baggage.

A person with a fever may seem absolutely flattened for weeks, and barely able to speak or lift their head off the pillow. This does not mean they are low in vital energy. Far from it; a good fever is evidence of good reserves. They are, in fact, expending it on a healing process. They will likely soon recover, more energetic, with fewer symptoms and better cheer, and seeming healthier all round. They will have used up some of their vitality in the process, but towards a valuable end, namely greater efficiency afterwards.

Even more subtle or chronic signs of ill health may be down to an incredible internal juggling act that is keeping the person alive. They may have plenty of vitality, they just don't have any spare for rock climbing or late-night dancing. Just because they aren't going to the gym every day, don't be quick to judge; they may be very wise not to.

Most of us know of people who seem to shine brightly for a while, yet only a few short years later, appear as shadows of their former selves. The fall after the rise does not necessarily mean they are completely drained of vital energy. They may have a great deal left, but it might now all be redirected to repairing the damage. Or it may simply be a better reflection of who they really are when they turn down the heat.

Most of us also know of people who, through determination, managed to overcome a dire illness, or to pull it all together to make it to a special occasion, or complete some long-planned project, and really shone for a while, only to be dead a few months later. These sorts of crashes and rapid declines may be a sign that they had been digging deeply within themselves, pressing the accelerator hard with a nearly empty tank.

We surely also know people who may seem very unhealthy for a time, or living unhealthy lifestyles, who one day, after turning things around, gain a new lease on life and become pictures of health. It is not that they have gained vitality, it is just that their output is no longer getting wasted. They can make highly worthwhile changes to their prospects, but what they can't do is get back what they have spent.

A truly healthy lifestyle, then, is one that uses our vitality sparingly whenever possible; and that when we do use it in bigger bursts, it is directed towards efficient productivity. And that includes being as creative as we are supposed to be, whether through our sport, or art, or raising children or building a business, or whatever.

Those things are also aligned with our survival and our reasons for being alive.

For practitioners, it is crucial to understand that we cannot increase our patient's vitality. We can only redistribute or reallocate what they have left, and we had better do so wisely. And in that regard, practically every therapy can be used in both positive and negative ways.

Therapies used unwisely can give an appearance of huge benefit while drawing down heavily on vitality in order to achieve it. Drugs are obvious examples, since they use poisons to achieve their effect, and so do some herbs. They do not work by removing stress. Rather, they alter the general equilibrium by applying an additional stress, so that the problem may manifest later or in some other way.

Following short-term use of a drug, its removal will generally allow the equilibrium to return to how it was before, providing no major permanent change has taken place. Of course, there is always change, and there will have been an expenditure of vitality due to the drug itself. But in somebody with adequate vital energy this will go unnoticed, in the same way that a mile driven on a full tank doesn't seem to matter as much as a mile driven when the tank is nearly empty, even though the fuel used is the same.

A treatment which appears superficially to be beneficial in youth can therefore be highly disruptive to somebody who is near the end of their natural life. Low vital energy is one way to explain why the elderly seem to suffer more problems from medication, with less benefit. Sometimes, the best thing to be done when hope has been lost is to take the person off all medication. Incidentally, only the prescribing doctor—or the patient himself—can do this. The mistake is to assume that the patient's decline is simply natural, and that the drugs aren't the problem. Tragically, when the stage is reached that medication is withdrawn, all life-supporting care, such as food and water, may sometimes be removed as well. Removing medical treatment as a last resort is completely reasonable, although selling the idea is a lot harder than it should be. But removing the basic needs of life from a vulnerable person is barbaric.

So-called natural therapies can also cause a considerable draw down on vitality. They can all, potentially, be used to remove inefficiencies, or to create them. But there must also be sufficient vital energy to withstand and process the treatment.

There are examples are in the dietary field, where one person may eat an all-meat diet to deal with an inability to handle vegetables and sugars, and another may go vegan to address a lack of willingness to eat meat. Restricted diets can liberate and divert energy that is otherwise tied up in digestion. This can give a sense of raised health and energy for a while; that is, until another bigger problem comes along, namely malnutrition. Once the internal reserves of essential substances are depleted, health can crash, or decline so gradually that the individual does not attribute it to the regime they are convinced is still doing them good.

I have known people who were adamantly wedded to strict and extreme diets that had for a while improved their sense of well-being, but that later on led to signs of diet-related illness. Yet resumption of a normal diet, even on a trial basis, was the very last thing they would consider. The right diet for someone at a particular time is not necessarily the right diet for every person for all time.

Examples in other fields are many. Isolated cracking of stiff joints without addressing general patterns of stress can free up one's mobility but lead to even greater rigidity before very long. The usual response is even more cracking until eventually no amount of skill can bring the same relief.

When a problem clears up through acupuncture, the effect can appear as magical. Most people don't even wonder where the energy for that has come from, yet it must have come from somewhere. Realistically, it has been diverted. The true cause is not a blocked meridian. The cause is the stress that meant the meridian had to be blocked. It only works if the stressful influence has been dealt with, otherwise the most it can achieve is costly palliation.

For the cranial osteopath or cranio-sacralist, soothing a disturbed cranial rhythm while leaving postural distortions in place can cause great confusion in a system. The effects on mind, body, and spirit can be insidious. Put simply, if somebody has twists and turns all the way up a lesioned spine, they *should* have a disturbed cranial rhythm and tension in the various membranes. Easing those things without addressing the mechanical lesion can cause a terrible disconnect that makes restoration harder, which I will explain later. The drain on vitality to keep achieving the sense of bliss each time can only be guessed at.

On the other hand, if the causal mechanical lesion is addressed then there is no reason that the functional disturbance should persist. Then those other interventions will be needed less and will work better. I am not saying cranial treatment is without usefulness, but—and like me or not for saying it—it is treating effects, not causes, and that is why I haven't personally developed my approach much along those lines. If it seems to be *needed,* then there is usually something else being overlooked.

I have met lots of people with chronic problems who have, through cranial treatment, become fairly comfortable within their situation but never moved beyond it, including devout practitioners of the art. If it is any consolation, there is no approach that is immune to this trap.

Homoeopathy's mechanism involves resonance between the patient and the remedy, meaning that a remedy is unlikely to do much harm—or much good—if it isn't the right match for the patient. But if the various internal, external, and lifestyle causes of the patient's stress are not understood then homoeopathy too will be limited.

It is quite possible for a psychotherapist to dismiss outright any idea of a somatic element to a patient's distress; still keeping them coming back twice a week for years. If the patient can afford it, then at least there is very little harm. In some cases it can be enormously helpful, particularly where trauma is severe, deep-seated or confusing. But for many it could be a case of keeping the patient amused while nature solves the problem (more on that later).

Similar critiques can be applied to most therapies. All have their uses, and all can add to the burden. But I must emphasise it is the therapist that matters and not the label.

It is no surprise then that we see patients becoming dependent on therapy, or their problems subtly escalating.

In practice, there is no therapy that can't gain something from occasional collaboration. But reductionism can hide behind modalities, and you can't tell just from the name of the therapy.

There are so-called osteopaths working in hospitals, but they can be osteopaths in name only, since they do not have a say in the general direction of care. Medicine's empty philosophy leads the way wholly. They get given a foot to treat, while drugs address the stomach or whatever. The kindest word I can use for this is physiotherapy.

The warning is that specialisms have a tendency to drain vitality, however the outcome may seem in the short term. Used judiciously they can get one out of a bind. And so, reductionism is not without some usefulness, particularly in emergency medicine. Temporarily drawing down on vitality to save life or achieve lasting healing is acceptable. Increasing the drain repeatedly in pursuit of a series of temporary results is not, and invariably the result is dependency. It can be a hard distinction to make, but it is a useful one, and vitality just gives us another way to look at it.

It took me a long time to understand that a natural therapy can cause these same negative progressions as pharmaceuticals, and had I not walked that walk towards complexity and dependency as a patient, I might not have learned to recognise it in practice either.

The first time I imagined my age was to blame for my own aches and pains, I was in my thirties. In fact, it wasn't the age, it was the miles. Had I not met a brilliant teacher, able to grasp this issue and explain it, who knows how I might have ended up? And had that same teacher not, over a year or two, helped me get on track, I wouldn't have known that there are better ways to do things, nor that greater resilience and less dependence overall could be achieved. I also did not expect the awkwardness and resistance I could meet when raising these discussions with patients and practitioners of all kinds.

Further reading

Dr Henry Lindlahr, book, *Philosophy of Natural Therapeutics.*

Missing Link 11: Constitutional diagnosis and treatment

Listen to your patient, he is telling you the diagnosis.

—William Osler

There is a medical joke, that diagnosis means translating the patient's symptoms into Latin. So, if you ask your doctor about an inflamed joint, he will reply, "You have arthritis."

Wonderful! People might think, to have their problem properly identified. The trouble is it doesn't tell you anything useful about the cause. It merely puts you in a bracket, which more often than not seals your fate.

It is often said that effective treatment begins with accurate diagnosis. But if we're serious about results, then what matters is *relevant* diagnosis, and the 'what' is usually not as relevant as the 'why'. And the why can sometimes be very imprecise and elusive.

By analogy, specific diagnosis describes a car crash and the wreckage that follows, while constitutional diagnosis is more about understanding the road, the car, the driver, and the chain of events that led up to the accident.

Whether the car bursts into flames or ends up on its roof, those things don't help us work out how to survive the next journey. What we really need to know is if the cause was a blind bend, a mechanical fault, or a distracted driver.

And medical treatment tries to fix the car, which would be reasonable if it were a car you were dealing with. But in a living body, the system can only heal itself, and it can't do that very well as long as the circumstances remain that promote the problem.

How many people take anti-inflammatories for arthritis, only to end up with worse inflammation as the body tries even harder to repair the joints? Inflammation (the *-itis* in arthritis) is our primary repair process. Treating it as if it were the primary cause of disease is what worsens the disease.

How many receive surgery and chemotherapy for cancer, only to find that more tumours pop up, sometimes much faster than the first one? A great many, I believe. In medicine, this is thought to be caused by metastasis; the cancer spread itself around the body because the surgery got there too late or missed a bit. What if the real reason was that the *cancer state* wasn't removed with the tumour? The body really needed that tumour as a dustbin for toxins, and when you cut it out, it has to make another tumour, and fast.

People might wonder how a terminal disease can be a survival mechanism. Ask Mother Nature, I suggest. My guess is that if you live another year and during that year you do something useful for your children, then that is an evolutionary advantage. If the toxins are instead left free-floating around the body, the chances are you will be dead much quicker. In support of this idea, when Max Gerson first put people on intensive juice diets for cancer, patients would sometimes die of liver failure due to the release of toxins from the disappearing tumours. Gerson Therapy progressed to include the coffee enema, which allows the liver to drain more effectively, in practice removing that problem.

Pursuit of causation could lead one into some quite complex reasoning processes, chasing causes from each link in the chain back to the one before. What tends to happen is the trail branches out as you follow it backwards, leading to many small causes, none of them critical on its own. The inflammation is caused by, say, five other things, and each of those is caused by five more, and so on. It's a bit like following one's family tree backwards to find out who one's true ancestors were. The answer is everybody and nobody. Hence, treating the cause sounds nice, but finding cause through an abundance of reductionism leads nowhere. The trail spreads out so thin and wide that soon there is nothing to follow. There has to be another way to get into it.

Medical diagnosis is concerned with the differences between conditions, while holistic diagnosis is concerned with the commonalities. For example, we are not trying to work out which of the many named varieties of arthritis may be causing the swelling in the joints. In that realm, you can ask different specialists and get different answers, spending months going from department to department. In the end, what you get is which painkiller to try first.

In reality, two people with exactly the same diagnosis can have completely different sets of circumstances. And two people with exactly the same circumstances—same job, adjacent desks, eating in the same canteen, living in the same neighbourhood, going to the same pub—can have completely different sets of symptoms. Medicine has no coherent and rational system for dealing with this, so it ignores cause at that level.

Try this for size: the notion of discretely identifiable diseases with distinct causes is a fallacy.

And when that philosophy fails to deliver the non-existent single cause, it steers medics towards the unmanageable parts of the problem for their excuses—genetics, old age, autoimmunity, viruses, and so on. It's all grist for the research mill but does little to deliver cures.

Florence Nightingale wrote that "there are no diseases, only disease conditions." Which brings us back to an earlier point, that the only workable solution to disease is health.

Holists are looking for common themes and patterns, and trying to understand which of those patterns could account for the symptoms, as well as any exceptional circumstances that come to light. Then they look to the aspects they can change, which is obviously where they should be looking.

When making a diagnosis, we need to understand roughly three main things:

1) The stress the patient is under;

2) The way their system handles that stress, including the adaptations it makes in order to cope; and,

3) The obstacles to recovery.

Opportunities for simple interventions lie in all three areas. Anyone can begin looking at the first, stress, and the more experienced we are, the more we can engage with adaptations and obstacles. These aren't strict categories and there is a lot of overlap. It doesn't really matter.

There may be no precise biological definition of the constitution, and different therapies handle it in very different ways. But this process of analysis is pretty much the basis of constitutional diagnosis.

Based on those three things, we devise our interventions. Our scope of practice is limited only by our creative ability in those areas and is therefore not precisely defined either. We can't look to statistical studies, since every case is unique, and so we are always dealing with a sample size of one. But what we do see are certain general patterns that come up again and again, meaning that in order to be useful, the amount of knowledge we need is less. In turn, constitutional approaches have an in-built tolerance of error, something we should look for at all times.

When we think of stress, we often think of emotional or mental stress, which in turn is rooted in external circumstances, past or present. We must look to our ways of coping, of course, but more importantly to the situations we face and how we deal with them. Wild animals find this easy. If a bird sees a cat, it flies off. There is no dilemma. But we humans see trade-offs for everything, and this is how we get into trouble. We might tolerate a toxic situation at work, for instance, in order to pay our bills. We end up using one kind of stress to offset another.

If we get better at this juggling act, life seems to get easier for us, and if not, life gets more complicated.

But stress means anything at all that creates work for the system. Most stressors are, in fact, physical, and so, the solutions will ultimately be practical. Inactivity and stagnation are a form of stress as well. Loss of direction is hugely detrimental, and something modern life can send in abundance. No wonder some people do literally want to fly away from their situations.

"But what can I do about it?" people very often ask.

It's true we can't always change our circumstances, and sometimes it is damaging to try. Step one is simply to map out the situation, even if we don't at first see a way through. Eventually, little opportunities for change will appear, and we will be better placed to take them. And sometimes acknowledgement of the problem is enough to summon the solution.

Of particular interest to osteopaths is postural stress. And I don't mean just standing badly, letting your shoulders droop. I mean the countless changes that take place in the micro and macro mechanics as we adapt to life's challenges, with all the resulting inefficiencies that can bring about. Their purpose is to save energy in the face of persistent stress, but as life goes on, we acquire a lot of redundant baggage.

Where the stress comes from is one thing, and how the body deals with it is another. Every chain has its weakest link, and something will suffer eventually if we keep loading it up. So, no matter how good we are at manipulating the body and its behaviour, we must never lose sight of the general loading on the system.

Machines have only one pathway for stress: they wear out and eventually break. But the body deals with stress in a great number of ways. It can resist it, it can absorb it, it can dissipate it, it can direct it somewhere, it can run away, and if it can't do any of those things, it can adapt to it. Stress can even strengthen it, but failing that, it can keep patching things up while waiting for a chance to get on top. Finally, it can fail under it, as well.

With only limited resources, the body has to prioritise. What is often called wear and tear is more accurately a case of insufficient repair to keep up with workload. As a temporary fix, crude thickening may shore things up, and stiffness, pain, fatigue, or other changes, may limit use.

The roughening around joint margins, for example, known as osteophytes, are the so-called pathological changes seen in arthritis. In a way, they are like calluses of the joints. They might slow or reduce erosion of the all-important joint tissue—articular cartilage. The inflammation is frantically trying to get on top of it all, even as we continue to work the structures through our daily lives.

So, we must consider the workload and the resources, and what else may be placing demands on those resources, before assuming degeneration is inevitable.

We also see stiffness and thickening in an artery. Low-density lipoprotein—cholesterol—patches up the damage caused by insufficient Vitamin C [1]. Those 'blockages' are actually the body's way of keeping blood flowing. It is only when the plaques are far advanced that the effects of narrowing are felt.

The actual heart attack is really an electrical or neurological event. Arteries are not passive tubes, like hosepipes. They are muscles. They squish and squash to regulate their own internal diameter, harmoniously adjusting the blood to all parts of the body according to demand. This takes place under direct control of the nervous system. Once again, it is when the body can't reconcile the demands with the resources that we get true structural or functional failure.

Chronically, this may manifest as heart failure (weakening of output). Acutely, however, a sudden increase in demand may outpace the response of the vessels. This is the classic model of angina and heart attacks.

But there is also the disturbance to the heart rhythm. Where does that come from? A build up of cholesterol doesn't account for it. The vascular constriction and fibrillation are features of a more general electrical disruption.

The heart itself is more like a valve than a pump. It is a great, spiral-shaped, mixing, whooshing structure with all kinds of far-reaching electrical properties. It maintains and regulates the natural momentum of the blood in coordination with many other structures. During a cardiovascular event the normal electrical symphony becomes a disordered cacophony.

Crucially, the disturbance to the regulatory mechanisms of the vessels, when faced with a sudden stress, may shut down the supply of blood to parts of the heart muscle itself.

Note the words: a disturbance to regulatory mechanisms.

This is one example of an acute problem that can kill you. But notice what the body is trying to do when it happens: it is trying to survive another threat. The failure comes after all other strategies for extended stress have done their very best.

The prior narrowing of the arteries, through those necessary plaques, is like a big handful of straws on the camel's back. But without them, who knows what might have happened, and much sooner?

The role of the structural lesion in this process was well established long ago [2] [3], and I can personally attest that this is not a mere academic matter.

I know people would who like nothing more than a chance to take this research further, and they would do it well. Even the medical mainstream catches a glimpse from time to time but has no idea what to do with it [4].

No doubt, the homoeopaths, naturopaths, acupuncturists, ayurveda practitioners, kinesiologists, and more, all have their own understanding of how the body prioritises resources, both over time and during immediate need. Pick any one of them and apply it, and you may well increase your chances of living longer and more comfortably.

As practitioners, we can redistribute stress and resources, but we must do so in a way that is energetically favourable overall, and some of the concepts in other chapters can help us with that. Even if wear, tear and damage seem unavoidable, we are still mindful that our bodies are finding the best possible balance under the circumstances.

So, what is the constitution?

Some might say it is our natural set of tendencies and responses. Others say it is the way in which the person's stress shows up.

A complete picture of the constitution also takes into account our patient's creativity and expression, and value system. He may be suffering for his art, but that is a part of his condition as well. Within the constitutional framework, we must still assume that the best balance is being achieved. And while a kind suggestion may be useful here and there, simply urging him to leave behind what matters in life can backfire. Without undertaking some more general work, a person who gives up smoking will quickly revert, or find another addiction. A new exercise programme won't last long.

Whether or not we can really change the constitution, or should, are big questions. And I suppose it all depends on our own personal definitions. The homoeopaths examine the character of the patient in some detail, as well as the health, trying to establish the individual constitution, and looking to influence it at an energetic level. I have seen homoeopathy change people's lives. The question is whether this really changes their constitution, or rather helps them work more effectively within it. When the chips are down is when the answer might be revealed.

This is a bit like gardening. A gardener can tend to the soil, taking into account the local conditions, and planting things that are appropriate and mutually supportive. Or he can bring in turf on a lorry, install half-grown shrubs, irrigating them and pouring chemicals around them to keep them alive. In healing, as in gardening, the direct approach may seem easier at first, but it makes more work sooner or later. To grow more exotic plants might require more technical gardening. And when the next storm comes through, the changes might be quickly undone. I suppose that the constitution is the set of local conditions that the gardener must always take into account.

Osteopathically, we are looking primarily at physical mechanics as our inroad. Within the posture, we can see sources of stress, patterns of its distribution, and obstacles to recovery, all woven together. And in theory they can, over time, be changed. In practice, not always—but they can usually be reduced.

But the body has a memory, which I will discuss later, and therapy can come undone somewhat in times of stress.

Perhaps, then, a good way to describe the constitution is as the body's memory of who we really are.

Constitutional diagnosis requires developing an understanding of general patterns: patterns of structure or function, or both, whatever is appropriate for the discipline. There are those patterns common to all of us, those unique to the patient in front of us, and those that have arisen out of the life the patient has lived. This does not by any means exclude what has just happened to them or which bit is hurting, but it cannot rest at that.

The homoeopath determines the constitution by interviewing the patient. The osteopath investigates the lesion by examining the global and local mechanics of the body. He tries to reconcile them with the physiological changes that are either observed or reported by the patient. While the lesion concept implies patterns of dysfunction, it is to a large extent integrated with healthy function as well. And in as much as treating the lesion pattern can enable the body to function more efficiently, it is essentially a constitutional approach.

Alas, modern osteopathy is far more linear and seldom invokes the constitution. The requirements of state regulation do place the emphasis on specific diagnosis and screening for pathology.

Around the time of my own training, there was increasing awareness of a disconnect between osteopathic philosophy and the teaching of clinical practice. Considerable effort was made to update the theory side of the curriculum to address this. Academic staff had to reapply for their own jobs.

The remit of the project was to make the philosophical training more relevant to clinic. Unfortunately, there wasn't a project to go the other way—to make clinic more relevant to osteopathy. Long before then, it was already well and truly 'medicine lite'.

Many natural therapies have their own version of the constitution, but whether or not that is invoked depends on the individual therapist. There are some therapies—and many therapists—seeming to lack a sense of the constitution, discarding anything not closely linked to the presenting complaint.

I know that homoeopathy has suffered the same problems as osteopathy, even without the carrots and sticks of regulation.

Mainstream naturopathy is very different now from the original nature cure movement. And I'm afraid, much of what I see there now is fighting disease with nutraceuticals. There may even be a subset of naturopaths hoping to control the market in vitamins, eventually. Those elements will welcome regulation until the true cost comes clear.

The point is that regulation and training have become a challenge to thinking about health on a constitutional level.

The expectations and demands of the patient can lead the holist into reductionism as well if we are not careful. Even when the patient seems strongly attached to their medical diagnosis, we should do our utmost to account for their problem in some other, more general way. Otherwise, we risk ourselves becoming just another part of the chronicity machine (more about that later). If the patient is determined to see their general therapist as a specialist, then the chances are they are missing the tapestry and seeing only the threads. Invariably, they will assign some other solution to many of the threads. The practitioner may not even realise that is what is happening. The patient may even control the therapy, what I call 'asking for highlights and tints'.

The important thing is to remain on course and not get drawn into errors of judgement through compromises made purely to please the patient. I have seen plenty work that way—trying to be all things to all people, saying the patient knows what they want. And it is inviting problems. It is far better for the patient to become dissatisfied and find somebody else than to be harmed because the practitioner gets led off course. Perhaps they will come back when they are ready ...

As a patient, it matters little what therapist you prefer so long as they can actually invoke a sense of context to your problem. But I would add that no therapy is likely to be complete without some respect for posture. It seems like common sense that if the wheel is wonky, the machine can't work properly until it is straightened; and moreover, that you can't drive the wheel straighter, as that only makes it worse. This may sound like an appeal to direct therapy. But it shouldn't, providing I have managed to convey the complex nature of the disturbances, that the wonky wheel represents.

The last point on diagnosis is about assessing chronicity, that is, the nature and degree of adaptation that has accumulated. Like vitality, there is an unavoidably high level of subjectivity in assessing chronicity, hence, a level of maturity and experience is helpful.

Understanding chronicity is vital not just for prognostication, but for tracking progress. Without understanding the chronic state, it is very hard to recognise whether or not the case is on track and to direct treatment accordingly.

Much as we all want our patient to get better as quickly as possible, one of the most terrible things we can do is to deepen their chronicity by taking shortcuts—by going straight for the problem area, the symptom, the proximate diagnosis, our favourite technique. The potential damage from doing so can go unrecognised—and even be interpreted as improvement—for a very long time. Approaching their problem from a constitutional perspective is one way to avoid this.

[1] Phillip Day, book, *Health Wars*, Credence Publications.
[2] Louisa Burns, film, *Heart Disease. Early Osteopathic Research by Louisa Burns DO,* https://www.youtube.com/watch?v=JW-OED7r6IY.

[3] A S Nicholas et al., *Randomised Controlled Trial, A somatic component to myocardial infarction*, British Medical Journal (Clinical research Edition) 1985 Jul 6;291(6487):13-7.

[4] *Blood pressure's a pain in the neck*, New Scientist, 11 August 2007.

Missing Link 12:
Patterns and how
they interact

The way is long if one follows precepts,
but short ... if one follows patterns.

—Seneca the Younger

Once you buy into the idea of non-linear treatment
and find ways to adopt it in practice, you get valuable
insights and results that are pleasing, though often confusing. This is especially so in complex or unusual cases,
where it may be unclear exactly what is going on at first.
In those cases, an indirect approach gives you plenty to
get on with that will be helpful, nevertheless.

In turn, the feedback you get from making those initial
inroads helps you to unravel more of the puzzle.

In contrast, direct therapy requires you to have it all
figured out before you begin, which can make it hard to
get going with an unclear case. This greatly increases the
importance of things you don't know.

One early result I had was a lady with sore thumbs,
where the cause was not one single obvious thing; a perfect candidate for a non-linear approach. About three

treatments were enough to remove the symptoms altogether, during which I never did anything to her actual
thumbs. I didn't hear from her again for a few months
until, one day, she called saying she had dropped a heavy
object on her foot, at which point, the pain in the thumbs
came back.

What this confirms is that the body has a memory.
There are certain patterns stored within the body into
which the system naturally retreats or collapses at the first
sign of stress. Hence, four colleagues doing similar work
may end a hectic week with completely different symptoms: the first gets a headache, the second gets a flare-up
of a stomach ulcer, the third will become anxious, and
the fourth will be doubled up with back pain. They may
all take completely different treatment, yet all are basically
variants of the same problem.

A disease-based model would consider them all as
completely different and, more than anything, this highlights the absurdity of specialisms. Additionally, it calls
into question the precisely defined scopes of practice
based on techniques, regions, systems, or other assumptions. The effective practitioner is concerned not with his
favourite conditions or techniques, but with the stresses
on the body, the obstacles to recovery, and whether or
not it is within his own creative ability to address those.

A question I avoided in an earlier chapter was to do
with how an osteopath treating a whole pattern in the
body can be getting any closer to treating primary cause
than by simply treating isolated segments, since the pattern
itself has causes. I hope to answer it here. The reason it
matters is that some believe the posture can be addressed

through very indirect means indeed, for example through the general unravelling that follows homoeopathy or craniosacral therapy. I don't believe it can in that way, at least not always. There are elements to the posture that those approaches cannot hope to address ever, since they are not acquired but inherent to our being and are therefore as close to primarily causal—or at least constitutional—as one can hope to get. Rather, it is the compressive effect of gravity exaggerating these patterns that leads to trouble, and, like the constitution in homoeopathy, that compression is often treatable without needing to look anywhere else.

I believe it is legitimate to say that structural osteopathy can—repeat can—address true cause, while therapy based around modifying the function can normally only treat effects. Osteopaths believe above all else—and I would say it is common sense—that structure governs function. The relationship between the two is consistent as long as function is not tampered with directly in isolation, in which case it seems some kind of decoupling can occur.

I have seen this happen in other areas of life, for instance, in synthetic parachute lines. Parachutists are supposed to untwist their brake lines after every jump. Leave it a few jumps and the lines will twist up to become noticeably shorter. But still, when you untwist them, they go back to normal. But if you keep flying the canopy with twists in place, subtly modifying the control inputs to compensate, something strange happens. The memory of the material eventually creates a new pattern, whereby the flat-braided tube acquires a spiral crease along its length. The result is an in-built spiral form, which the more you try to untwist, the more it seems to twist up the other way. It is bizarre, but the end result is there is no way to untwist the line: all you can do is choose which of the non-ideal twists seems better. Eventually, you have to change the lines.

The human body does the same thing, in that when you train it through discipline or therapy to function in the presence of a structural lesion, you can make it comply, but then there is no way to unravel the structure without winding up the function. This is the decoupling I mean. What you get is a patient who is very well adapted to a disturbed situation, but who is not in a state of ease when everything is right with the world.

A physical manifestation of this might be the scoliosis, where the spine is at its most neutral when twisted. Similar principles can show up in the mental and social realm, where somebody who has lived through an abusive situation will no longer function fully in a supportive environment, and may unconsciously seek out difficulty, perhaps ending up in a series of unhealthy relationships.

When, through physical therapy, the patient starts getting used to how true postural ease feels, they begin to notice more clearly the stresses that are causing them pain and can quickly respond to them more effectively. In this way, I have seen people change their habits without my having to make assumptions about their problems. They begin to see workable ways through previously insurmountable situations. On the other hand, creating a sense of ease within those situations can leave the patient stuck in them forever. They can then become resistant to any therapy that offers real change. This is why an emphasis on palliation can cause lasting limitations to prospects.

You can often tell when a patient is really getting better because their problem seems to simplify. Their symptoms become localised, and sometimes more intense at the same time. Many will at first think this means they are getting worse, but it usually moves on from there quite quickly. Their vague troubles seem to take a more definite form. The nagging low back ache becomes a sharp pain whenever they move in a certain way, and they know what to do differently. The patient who used to live under a cloud of misery now starts talking about why they hate their job. The emotional becomes the mental and so on (Hering's Law).

There is an insidious side to some of the more fluid-based cranial and visceral manual techniques, which I will try and make clear. They can be helpful if the cause is a partially resolved trauma; say, a blow to the head, or damage while giving birth. The problem comes when these functional techniques are applied without an awareness of structure or of general patterns. And this is what leads to the sort of decoupling I just described.

Chemical, fluid, cellular, mental, and energetic therapies that otherwise deny the primary importance of physical structure are always limited, in my view. I have cases overseas where a lot can be done without being physically present. Usually though, a point is reached where it is necessary to deal with the posture. If others say they can do a complete job entirely through functional approaches, then good luck to them, but it does seem to me like treating effects before causes.

I accept that posture is influenced by organic health as well as the other way around, and that all kinds of therapies can work in mysterious ways. But metaphysics can quickly become a hiding place for those who lack an eye for actual physics.

There are those who would say that no, we rest on consciousness, or light, or energy. To an extent, I can go along with that. But so what? When I meet someone who has been through functional, energetic or metaphysical therapies for an unresolved problem with a clear set of physical drivers, I can't help thinking something fundamental has been overlooked, especially if the results are unimpressive. It happens.

As I said earlier, if there is a pattern of physical stress in the body, then the function *will* be disturbed. The cranial-rhythm will not be smooth. There will be tension in the membranes. There will be knock-on effects on the organs. These are fundamentals. Smoothing the cranial ebb and flow, easing the tension, 'supporting' the organs, or otherwise tampering with the internal economy of the body, while overlooking the postural lesion, is to cement an altered relationship between signal and response. It takes the system out of its lowest energy state. The clues to this are that the problem seems to become more complex and confusing, and the patient, who wants nothing more than a thorough solution to his problem, becomes dependent on therapy. He risks being led on long journeys into other realms in search of far-off breakthroughs.

Unwillingness to face this huge issue is a real blind spot for the modern osteopathic profession. Rather, it attempts to go deeper by taking a more cranial, visceral, or naturopathic direction, while at the same time presenting to the world an acceptable but much shallower musculoskeletal front, then recombining it all as some kind of proxy for holism. Others may attack me for this. They are free to state their case, and I hope they do. We urgently need to have these discussions without falling back on theoretical physics, huge deductive leaps, or distinct umbrage. What is generally missing from these conversations is a willingness to set the terms, since at that point, the goalposts would have to sit still. The one and only thing that seems to unite osteopaths is the inability—more often than not absolute refusal—to agree on what is meant by osteopathy.

Some postural patterns may be inherently programmed into our being, and in that sense, they are as close to causal as we can get. Even so, we do not need to resign ourselves to their influence. In fact, we have little choice but to address them. They may at times be latent but become manifest or exaggerated under stress. If that is so, then we can be said to be addressing the cause by helping the posture back towards a more neutral state. The same principle may well apply in other therapeutic fields, but it is for others to explain them.

John Wernham put in a lot of work to understand a primary pattern that is always there, in all of us. What he actually stated was that it is *usually* there. But I have a sense he was talking from a practical position, and that in fact the reasons for the pattern are biological fundamentals, like having a heart on the left and a liver on the right. Some of us do have organs the other way around, but I have personally encountered only one definite example in twenty years of practise.

The question I have about primary patterns in other disciplines is whether they would offer such a clear practical handle as this one. The postural primary pattern may be no more or less a part of our innate being as anything, yet there are clear ways it can be approached without going against our nature. In treatment, we do not compensate for it, as that would add another stress. And nor do we alter it. Rather, its exaggeration from stress is reduced.

What makes the primary pattern so confusing is that it is combined with other patterns. I see roughly four general types. Trying to separate them all out in each and every patient would drive us mad. But for the sake of exploring a concept, separation can be a useful academic exercise. Ultimately, we have to put it all back together.

There is the immediate or acute pattern that results from stress or simply going about our day. When we pick up a heavy object, we change shape immediately to support it and keep our balance at the same time. This is not a static pattern, and we shift constantly as we hunt for ease. The heavy object is merely illustrative, since we are always changing shape, heavy object or not.

Then there are the adaptive patterns we get from sustaining or repeating something, and these involve structural changes at a tissue level—that is, some actual remodelling of the body takes place. The more time we spend in one shape or another, with or without some kind of loading, the more entrenched the adaptation gets. While we sit in a chair, we are not getting out of shape. Rather, we are getting in great shape for sitting in chairs. If we lift weights, we get in shape for that, but then I see plenty of weightlifters who hurt themselves just sitting on the sofa.

Injury spans those two other kinds, immediate and adaptive. We may walk with a limp from the pain of a leg injury, get a twist in the pelvis from it, even ending up with one leg positioned to be shorter than the other. Mental injury and stress also have postural effects, since posture contains mechanisms for protective behaviour as well as adjustment for our sensory attention. Posture is also a canvas for expression, which is why two practitioners can sometimes see the same patient quite differently. As far as postural patterns go, neither injury nor mental stress need their own categories: immediate and adaptive still suffice.

The important thing to see is that myriad causes from our actions, habits, and environment can imprint those patterns. And the patterns are always different and always changing. The immediate arises quickly, and it usually goes away quickly without much help. The adaptive arises more slowly and resolves more slowly, and it doesn't always resolve spontaneously.

The primary or general pattern mentioned earlier is always there and is pretty consistent. The only thing that changes much within a given individual is the degree to which it is expressed, which is a function of stress and gravity. And of course, we can make longer term adaptations there as well if we have to.

There is the possibility of another kind of pattern, and this one is more to do with who we actually are as individuals. It may to a degree be passed on, since I often see distinct postural features show up in a parent and all the children, and they can seem to run in families.

We have mentioned the constitution, which means our own unique set of tendencies that are somewhat independent of the lives we live. They are the bit we can't change just by eating right or exercising more, meaning they are truly constitutional.

In Ayurveda, dietary and lifestyle changes are used to balance the constitution, but as far as I know, this does not actually alter it. The changes must be sustained or else the situation will revert, perhaps during a time of heightened stress. Presumably this approach helps ... providing it is within the patient's constitution to stick with the programme.

Irony aside, therefore, constitution does affect how we deal with situations and make choices, so there are knock-on effects into precisely how we adapt. Put another way, people will form different kinds of adaptation to the same kind of stress. One will learn to talk his way out of situations, another will learn to punch his way out.

If, at this point, I've lost you, that's okay, and it doesn't matter that much if these are definitions that everyone will agree on. The point to understand is that there is not just one pattern, but a resultant of several patterns; that what we see in our patient is a summation of various influences, and this can really confuse us when we make our assessments. It is understanding that there is one definite pattern somewhere in amongst it all, which helps us to sort it all out.

One other point that needs stating is that all patterns—however we choose to categorise them—are not limited to the postural field. Our lesion, for want of a better word, is an entire multi-dimensional tapestry. Where and how to start tidying it up without pulling things apart is the conundrum. There are a few more insights that can save us here, and I will come to those.

Postural compression or collapse is comparable to the ways various different springs compress under a load. A spring usually compresses in a fairly elastic way, in that it returns to the same shape afterwards. The posture also has a degree of plasticity to it, like putty, meaning it does not return completely by itself, and this is what makes it a useful area of treatment—there is something we can help reverse.

Some of us compress or collapse in a lateral or rotational pattern, some of us in a forward and backward way, and there can be a focus in one place or another. This is a gross oversimplification, of course, and nothing happens in isolation.

Knowing that there are limitless unique combinations of many patterns ought to make a reductionist approach a real headache. You might not have heard of Fourier Analysis, or Fourier Transforms, unless you are an electrical engineer or a musician. Fourier Transforms are mathematical techniques for combining waves to make any waveform you choose. When you put together pure sine waves of different wavelengths and amplitudes, you always get a resultant wave that is a new shape. This is basically what an electronic synthesiser does in music. By combining many sine waves you can make literally any shape you want—a sawtooth, a square, a wave that is only peaks or only troughs, a wave that increases or decreases in amplitude over time, waves that have a beginning or an end with nothing before or after, a single spike, a wave shaped like a house or a car or the Eiffel Tower if you want, or a wave that appears completely random and never repeats. In music, you can make the sound of a trombone, or a bucket of coal tipped into a bathtub. You can make all these and many more out of multiple pure sine waves. The only limits are in the electronics, your imagination, and the ability to do the mathematics.

The extension of this principle to patterns of all kinds is that when you combine them, you can end up with resultant patterns that look quite unlike any of the component patterns. What you think you see may not be what is really there. Important features can hide.

Several important and useful points arise from this for treatment, and for bodywork in particular. A twist to the left may in fact be nothing to do with a group of muscles you identify as pulling things in that direction. That tight muscle may be stabilising the change instead of causing it. Some of the underlying patterns may be the exact opposite of what you see. So, you can't always treat what you see.

When the spine is in a comfortably neutral position, a rotation or a side-bend will normally involve all relevant segments moving in unison. When the spine is out of neutral, the same movement will cause some of those segments to move in the opposite direction, that being the only way the system can resolve the various forces involved. Increase the movement and the spine will tend to buckle at those segments, at which point protective mechanisms take over to prevent injury. We may feel this as pain or resistance, and this is often what sends us to the osteopath. Other structures may be recruited to compensate or protect, causing an antalgic posture (meaning avoiding pain), which is an overall lean or shift to spare the stressed area from further stress. Hence, the patient with a very acute back may be stooped or side-bent and complain that they are unable to straighten up.

Sometimes, the worst thing we can do then is to go directly to the tight bits and loosen them off, and just as bad is to force the whole body straighter. When specific adjusters observe, say, a 'flexion-sidebend-rotation' strain at a spinal segment, they need to be really careful not to stuff things up by simply correcting it, as that can disturb a complex global arrangement that specifics simply do not take into account. When the system gets really wound up, it may appear as if, for instance, one half of the pelvis is rotated forward and the other rotated backwards, when in fact there is a crucially important component pattern going the other way.

When I met Mr Wernham a few weeks before he died, he put to us a question about what he called the mystery of the short lateral curve. Basically, this is a localised disturbance in an otherwise apparently normal spine. "What is it, and what causes it?" he asked.

At the time, none of us could answer it. I am sure now that the answer lies in a combination of global patterns that produces no obvious general shape change but leaves a clear trace in one small region. It can even appear as if a single segment has jumped out of line for no reason.

If this deceptive combining effect is not understood in treatment—as it so often isn't—then harm can be the result of the supposed corrections.

I'm afraid I don't have much sympathy for the highly goal-centred and linear approach of some exercise-based interventions. If something is too long, work it to tighten it. If something is too short, stretch it, and so on. It can pay dividends for a while. But invariably, new patterns are introduced making the whole situation even more complex, until the patient can't keep on top of all the exercises required to fix all the new manifestations. After a year or so, they are exhausted.

Some neuromuscular exercise theories claim to go deeper, through retraining the altered patterns of movement that stem from the disturbed postural mechanics. Chronic mechanical patterning issues certainly can arise from lack of free movement in the infant, leading to poor coordination. But it's a leap too far to say that improving coordination through discipline can somehow rework the development. It is too late. The level of micromanagement and control-freakery of that approach flies in the face of belief in a self-righting system with innate intelligence that always knows what it is doing.

If the profile of the spinal arches is disturbed, then coordination will be disturbed, and moving differently in the hope of correcting the spine takes a lot of mental effort for very little reward. Even basic core stability approaches miss the crucial point: healthy core muscle activation is essentially reflexive, i.e., automatic. We have the association all the wrong way around. You don't get a problem spine sorted by activating core muscles. You get the core muscles activating properly by sorting out the spine. Once again, you can't correct faulty wheel alignment by driving the car.

If there is a way to address one's own lesion effectively through movement, then it more likely comes through inquisitive self-exploration over a long period of time, than through pre-determined and goal-centred discipline. There are some systems that claim to approach things in that way.

And all the same points could be made about other fields besides postural mechanics. The osteoporosis example mentioned in Missing Link 7 (Chaos: complexity and non-linearity) is a good illustration. There we see interacting, the effects of diet, digestive inefficiency, indoor-living, waste retention, mental and physical stress, breathing patterns, all resulting in an increased need to draw minerals into the blood. What we think we see is a lack of calcium. So, the patient is given calcium tablets, and it doesn't work.

In another patient with the same set of challenges, their constitution will produce repeated urinary tract infections instead. Once again, their issue is not lack of antibiotics. We can easily bring the structural lesion into all this if we want, and sometimes we have to.

And thus, we see the commonalities between patient presentations, mentioned in the last chapter. The solutions require us to see general patterns in life, and to know our patient, rather than to learn every possible detail about thousands of separate diseases.

When there is so much possible confusion in assessing our patient, it is understanding that there are some

universal patterns in the body that gives us hope. Whatever we see, whatever the patient's body appears to be
doing, there are some things we know it must be doing,
even if it seems to be doing something else. If we can
understand some of the component patterns, then we
can look past the deceptive resultants to some extent.

Structurally, there is always—or nearly always—one
component pattern underneath that we know about, even
if we can't always see it, because it is (nearly) always there.

If we examine the body in the right way, we can get
enough clues to confirm its presence, and it offers us
some kind of solid starting point we can get onto. The
more it is hidden from us, the more we need to rely on it.
By unravelling the primary pattern with a general (non-
specific) approach, we can get some slack into just about
any situation. The other patterns often then become
more clear. The patient's shape may look worse for a
time but is in fact simpler to deal with. They may become
super aware of every imbalance, but eventually this feeling goes, and they regain freedom in their body. They will
even, out of nowhere it seems, start mentioning subjects
that are important to the next stage of recovery.

In the very acute cases with severe antalgic stoops, I
frequently see the patient look temporarily more wonky
at the end of the initial treatment, yet they report great
relief and can get their shoes on by themselves.

In the more general healing realm, the person with the
internal trouble may end up with new symptoms before
the main trouble goes away; for example, when digestive
issues resolve after a day of diarrhoea. What is going
on there? I believe the effect of reducing more general

stress gives the body enough slack to deal with the real problem, the toxic state. The resources required had previously been tied up with various—more immediately apparent—compensatory mechanisms.

Importantly, I very seldom work on the site of symptoms until it has regained enough resilience to accept the treatment. By then, more specific treatment often isn't needed, anyway. The converse, treating specifically at first, seldom deals with the more general state: it usually just pushes the problem around. Unlike some of my colleagues, I will never push the patient through pain, since the risks are far too high, in my view. Great caution is therefore needed if the patient is under the effect of painkillers during treatment.

Does this work in every case? 100% success would be implausible, but it works impressively often. When it doesn't, it usually means there is some additional unknown driver yet to be addressed. The point, about multiple patterns combining in deceptive ways, remains. Whichever way we develop our ideas in the future, I see great potential in recognising this issue.

The other not-so-secret weapon on which this all depends is the ability of the human system to recover when it is given a chance. The reduction of stress, from making inroads to the global patterning thus, means the system can start the actual healing. Remember that healing isn't what we do in treatment; it is what the patient does afterwards.

Missing Link 13: Gravity

Gravity is one variable in a lot of scientific processes. If you can remove gravity or minimize its effect, then you can understand the other processes that are going on.

—Laurel Clark, astronaut

There is plenty of debate about the nature and causes of gravity, but there is no denying its constant presence. In a sense, it kills us all in the end. But we also can't live well without it. Our entire evolution has taken place around its dictates. Every other aspect of our environment changes over time, whether quickly or gradually, even the cycles of night and day; but our relationship with gravity has, for aeons, been unwavering.

Our physical structure is a reflection of this inescapable force on us. Our perception depends so much on a clear sense of up and down that we work constantly at keeping our eyes and ears horizontal whenever possible, and when we can't establish a clear level, we can become disoriented, agitated, and even physically sick. And the physics that keeps us alive depends on our relationship with gravity, from the balance of pressures in our various cavities and the valves in our veins, to the size of our muscles and bones. The circulation of fluid, the removal of waste, and the pattern of our gait are all tuned to it.

Atmospheric pressure depends on gravity and with that, the function of our lungs, our breathing apparatus, and the exchange of gasses in our alveoli.

We have important homoeostatic functions to stop us from fainting when we stand up from a chair. We do not feel very well if we hang upside down for a while. We feel fear if we are high above ground and security when we are down on the earth. We could live on a planet that was lighter or heavier than ours, but the set-up would be badly out of tune and our health would be affected. Our bodies have been intricately organised to keep us on good terms with gravity, and from the moment of conception to the day we die, this involves a considerable energetic expenditure.

Furthermore, defiance of gravity is an important defining feature of multicellular life—possibly *the* defining feature—and one that isn't mentioned in textbooks. There is nothing that can actually direct itself to oppose gravity except living things and the devices we create. It seems wrong to ignore its importance in health and disease.

But because gravity is constant, and there is nothing we can do to change it, it gets overlooked almost completely in a healing context. I say almost always, because we all know to lie down to rest, flotation tanks are used for their relaxing effects, and it can be very relieving when pregnant or injured to go for a gentle swim. Hospitals use rebound stockings in those who are very immobile to help blood return from the legs. And in first aid, the importance of elevating parts of the body is known. But systematically directing gravity's influence as a means to raising health is not something in most practitioners' repertoires.

Gravity is so constant and universal that I would have overlooked it completely had I not caught myself mentioning it already. Bodyworkers ought to have an awareness of gravity, since in dealing with posture, we are inevitably dealing with a structure that must remain efficiently free-standing. Chronic disturbance of postural equilibrium can raise energetic demands considerably, long before it gets so severe that we are consciously aware of it. But bodywork when practised in a direct or linear way often overlooks this, and often amounts to finding all the tight or misaligned elements and then loosening them off or pushing them into line, without first considering why they have needed to be tight or misaligned, in the first place. The reason is gravity.

The physics of posture are complex and pretty poorly understood. Localised disturbance can be a necessary response to a more general disturbance, and vice versa. When we tamper with these local adaptations in isolation, we can easily invite in a more general collapse pattern, sometimes resulting in the sorts of slumped postures and drooping shoulders easily mistaken for just a sheer lack of discipline. Worse, we can create a need for a more severe adaptation and thus take the body out of its lowest energy state, leading to stuck joints, tension in the muscles, and increased demands for energy. For sure, rubbing a tight muscle can bring relief for a while. But if that muscle happens to be bracing the Leaning Tower of Pisa, and we do not address the lean, then at best it will only become tight once more. At worst, overall stress will increase and the patient moves that much closer towards disease.

Muscles are highly responsive and provide the body with immediate adaptation. They do not generally need us to change them. If they are tight, then it is because the body needs them that way. The intervention may be well-intentioned, but the supposition is that the tight muscle is causal and not the body's best solution; or that the misaligned vertebra is simply malfunctioning on its own. Were practitioners to see that relieving a sore muscle or cracking a joint could lead eventually to a diseased organ, they wouldn't dare touch them. But who can prove it?

So, there is a large amount of deniability built in, and many would happily carry on rubbing and cracking the same backs, sometimes for decades, even as the health visibly worsens, without any awareness that their own therapy is sickening the patient. So-called maintenance treatment for degeneration is often just that—it maintains the degeneration.

The smart way to soften a tight muscle and loosen a stuck joint—and keep them that way—is to remove the stress from them, so that movement becomes more useful to the body than rigidity.

Health-based therapies can't afford to overlook structural adjustment *as it relates to overall posture and gravity*. Treating biology as purely chemical—or cellular, energetic, mental, fluid etc.—is incomplete. And even combining all those elements isn't enough unless gross mechanical structure and posture are considered. It also isn't good enough adding on bodywork as a separate therapy 'for the structure'. So many dysfunctions that seem to be chemical or cellular—even psychological or infective—can derive from adaptations to gravitational stress, that in some cases they can be resolved by bodywork alone. If that were not the case, osteopathy would never have become a word.

I have seen bodywork quickly resolve chronic urinary tract infections, gut parasites, constipation in babies, blocked ears, heart disturbances, complex neurological issues and much more—without any other adjunctive measures, not even cranial or visceral work. All coincidence, of course! Actually, I can't always explain it, but how much in life can be explained, really?

In some cases, gravity is the only significant stress we can identify that hasn't already been exhausted as an inroad. Arguably, it should have been the starting point all along.

I used to visit an osteopath in England when my digestion was grumbling, and he would see me when his heart was fluttering. We never sat debating whether bodywork was the answer, we just got on with it. This was just another day at work for us.

Hopefully, this explains why I believe osteopathy deserves to live on, even though I have reservations about the direction the field has taken. I didn't begin with a background of bodywork, as many of my colleagues did. I began with a difficult problem to solve in my own life, and on the way came to realise there was no complete solution without understanding structural adjustment. And unlike the fields of diet, supplements, psychology, exercise, and all the rest that now are all well mapped out,

I found very little systematic guidance about the broader physiological effects of treating the structural lesion, even from the supposed masters of bodily manipulation. One time, I even got into trouble with the clinic faculty simply for asking about it.

The problem is that turning a blind eye to those effects doesn't make them go away; all it does is remove our ability to handle them.

At the time, many in the profession seemed happy practising a form of physiotherapy, made good livings from it, and sought to reach higher levels within that realm. Some did believe in more, but at best their theories were vague or inaccessible. They often drifted into the quantum, or even the metaphysical, when osteopathy is supposed to be practical above all else. They usually offered a collection of impressive techniques that were potent in their own way, but their explanations could leave a feeling of needing more. Hence, it all seemed like rumours and myths, and our college never offered us anything concrete.

This is not to criticise my college, which unquestionably still strives for excellence within the constraints given, merely to say that my own world view became increasingly at odds with those constraints. It was only after I graduated that I met people with a solid enough grip to make these ideas practicable. And healing should be practicable or else we've missed the point entirely.

Since gravity is so unavoidable—and since our relationship with it is so important, and since the body has in-built ways both to cope with gravity and suffer under it, and since it can only be aided significantly by deliberate input—gravity is as close to a clearly identifiable primary cause of disease as we can ever hope to get. Those other clear primary causes, such as injury, poisoning, malnutrition, physical and mental stress, all vary from case to case. Like any lifestyle or environmental factor, they need addressing. But gravity is universal. We know it is there, we know it is happening, we know where it leads, and we know how to relieve it in almost every case. We do not usually need to know all the ins and outs of why the posture has become wound up through compression, in order to know that the patient needs unwinding, and that only good can come of it.

As far as methods go, there are plenty of ways to ease the effect of gravity. A good night's sleep in a decent bed (without memory foam), flotation, gentle swimming, and my favourite, hanging from a bar, can all be very relieving, at least temporarily. But they can also work haphazardly. The relief they achieve may be partial or uneven, or towards some other pattern that isn't entirely neutral. Yoga, carefully practised, can have lasting effects, and is a powerful form of self-help. But seeing two people doing a downward dog side by side, you can't tell who is practising yoga and who is doing stretching exercises. Therefore, it is a good idea to read up on the theory of yoga or get help from a good teacher.

Great care needs to be taken with yoga when there are developmental or strongly adaptive issues, since the unwary can travel further into a dysfunctional pattern and believe they are doing themselves a lot of good.

Treating yogis can raise some curious concerns of its own. It can be hard to see what is going on, sometimes, since whatever is going on, they can be very good at controlling their posture. It can take a bit of work before one even sees the real patterns.

For the therapist, there are plenty of techniques to choose from, and the vast choice suggests that the method doesn't matter as much as the awareness and vision of the practitioner. But it is very easy to achieve superficial relief by going further into the lesioned pattern and away from an easy neutral.

For example, I have seen many patients with super straight or hyper-extended thoracic spines who had been advised to lie over foam rollers to extend their spines even further. It can take a while to impress upon a foam-roller user that the thoracic spine needs its curve, that being dead straight there is not healthy, and that the rigidity and pain have arisen from maintaining the extended posture. Taking an extreme situation, and making it more extreme by this exercise, is not helping.

Therapy, when misused, can simply break up presenting patterns instead of reducing them, allowing a new lesion to find its way in. The old bit stops hurting and a new bit starts. They say it brings relief at the time, but at best, it stops working sooner or later.

A sensible approach begins with a sensible idea of what a neutral posture should look like. There are ideals to which nobody conforms completely. But when we have a clear sense of neutral, then the disturbances can more easily show themselves to us. Being closer to neutral can't in itself do the patient any harm, so long as the method of getting them there is safe: that is, with due clinical awareness and without invoking undue force or pain. We may not move them very far towards neutral, but that is better than taking them in the wrong direction. And usually, a little is all it requires.

All of that could be a long course of study on its own. Since this book is not about precise adjustment theory and technique, the best I can say here is that the issues are real and need considering when undertaking training. If we don't take account of global patterns and the fact that they can interact, then we risk enhancing some of those patterns inadvertently.

So, we must look, firstly, at the patterns that we know are there underneath it all. We do at least understand (I believe) there is a primary pattern common to pretty much all of us, right down to a molecular level. Our apparent symmetry is illusory; an evolutionary fix that belies our actual development. We are even built of molecules (collagen) that have a spiral nature, making some kind of spirality our most efficient neutral state. It also sets the path for compression or collapse, and therefore has some influence on our adaptations to stress. Every dancer, every gymnast, every person who uses hand tools knows this, at some level.

Wernham's system of Body Adjustment, developed for more than half a century, took this into account. He produced a practical approach that deals with the entire primary pattern of compression and fully integrates the adaptive patterns at the same time. It guides the body towards neutral as far as it is willing to go without force, and doesn't give it space to drop further into the lesion pattern. The process is iterative; treatment-wait-response, treatment-wait-response, and so on.

Some practitioners believe they should never impose their will upon the patient's body, and that they should allow the body to tell them where it wants to go. I would counter that having a clear idea of what the body needs and guiding it there with consent is not imposing: it is the sort of competent clarity the patient is paying for. Practitioners who refuse to allow in such ideas as ideal normality and neutrality also don't like being told they lack any kind of goal to aim for, but if the hat fits, they can wear it. Allowing the patient's body to set the direction of therapy can be dangerous, since it can readily seek ease by retreating further into lesion. The result can be the situation getting worse underneath. The practitioner can end up dancing around the patient's dysfunction, and even sometimes picking up all their symptoms.

I am not saying that Wernham's system is the only valid system there is. I am saying it is one of the few I have encountered, that can bring together all my understanding of anatomy, physiology, complex systems, gravity, ethics, health and disease, and fit it all into a viable training and business structure. And his results were certainly impressive. Some of his students have gone on to advance his work in important ways. But none have successfully done so simply by introducing more techniques, or by changing the theory. They have done so by developing their understanding of the various adaptive patterns and of the body's basic needs. Those who have tried it and decided it doesn't work seem to have all made the mistake of thinking they could improve it by incorporating modalities.

One final word on gravity, and why it is such an important area in practice, is on the plasticity of the human body. We compress like springs, but to an extent, also like putty. In other words, if compression is sustained, we do not fully return to our original shape. Or, when we do bounce back, it is slow. It takes all night for us to regain the height we lose during the day. Repeated or sustained stress therefore has a chance to accumulate. The plastic aspect needs active measures to reverse it, without which tissues will eventually restructure themselves to function better as their compressed version. Some things will distort, others will shorten, thicken, harden, fibrose, or fuse.

Even bones will eventually take on new shapes as part of the adaptive process. Reversing that may be possible through the natural turnover of bone structure with time, but it is certainly slow.

Because elasticity is the greater part, we are not always aware of the plastic aspects. But they are there, and however tiny, their changes can become embedded more chronically, making survival that bit harder, and the reversal that much lengthier a process. Even if it is not to be reversed, its progression may be slowed, and there are always the less permanent changes to address before they become established.

Missing Link 14: The mental side and the influence of others

Do not adjust your mind, the fault is in reality.

—Ronald David Laing, Scottish psychiatrist

The role of the mind in physical and mental disease could fill a whole library; in fact, it already fills many libraries. So, it might not seem like a missing link at all. But it needs a mention here because I believe we have been led in completely the wrong direction with this. Our minds have become the front line in an ongoing political struggle, where information is a weapon.

There is little doubt that the mind and body have a strong influence on each other, and treating psychology as a separate discipline would not be holistic. Nevertheless, the general healer shouldn't be attempting to play psychotherapist, and for the most part it isn't helpful to try. But how we think about our situation does have a direct influence on our journey through health and disease.

What is easily overlooked is the inbound pathway in the mind-body symbiosis. By that, I mean, the influence of the body on our mind. It should be obvious that if our thinking is dysfunctional, it is not because the brain has simply gone and miswired itself, or that all our problems stem from that. There is increasing recognition of a gut-brain connection, but the immediate responsiveness of the mind to every part of the body, through direct neurological feedback, perhaps seems less obvious than it should.

For the therapist, the message is: whatever you think is going on with the mind, do *something* for the body and its environment. And I'll spend much of this chapter explaining why.

Still, it is much more useful to the powers that be that we do not see the great deal that is wrong with the world under their leadership, and that we believe instead that all our problems have somehow bubbled up inside of us for no reason.

I see various forms of this doctrine embedded in medicine: when science fails to help the patient, it is due to the flawed body and mind simply going wrong, rather than the perfect human form still suffering.

So, if we struggle to deal with the world, then supposedly it is our attitude that needs correcting, or even our brain chemistry, whether in school, or work, or prison, or in a social work context.

No doubt some people's attitude is problematic. But without a realistic sense of perspective and development of healthy boundaries all around, it may be hard even to fathom who really has the problem—the patient, the therapist, or even society. We have been gaslit, in other words (or gaslighted). And if the term 'gaslighting' isn't familiar, then there is an urgent need to catch up.

Gaslighting refers to when a person or group tries to gain power over another by presenting them with a distorted version of reality. The victim often feels they cannot trust their own senses and struggles to tell what is true and what is false. Just as likely, they do not even realise they are being controlled, and accept the authority of the other, believing them to be right. The term originates in the 1944 film, *Gaslight*, where a woman is made to feel as if she is going mad by her criminal husband, and even becomes isolated from the people who are trying to help her. Whole societies fall victim to gaslighting. The fact is we can hardly turn on the television or open a newspaper without being manipulated.

For those who have been affected—which means most of us—a great resource is David Gillespie's book, *Taming Toxic People* [1].

The paradox is that the disempowerment this causes, makes it very easy to see no solution other than the world and everyone else in it needing to sort themselves out. Obviously, that gets us nowhere. Or we ask for help, and the danger is that the help towards which we are directed is controlled more or less directly by the same forces that have created the mess to begin with. Our friends, families, and therapists are often as gaslit as we are.

When we start to get glimpses of the truth, we can find ourselves deeply divided from people we thought we could trust. Individuals can turn on each other instead of on an illegitimate authority, and one can easily retreat back under the illusions in order to avoid conflict. Help is out there, but we have to be very selective indeed. Hence, we still have no choice but to look inside ourselves to figure out what to do about the world outside.

It is no wonder then that some people hesitate to ask for help: or that in trying to escape hopelessness they may sabotage things with sudden bursts of misplaced action.

But increasingly, the vogue is that we have created our own reality entirely by our thoughts, that changing our mindset is what really matters, and that meditation, prayer, self-hypnosis, affirmations, spirituality, or straight-forward positivity will fix it. Fair enough, those things can be the beginnings of the journey. But it leads us nowhere unless at some point we can make hard decisions and take tangible real-world actions that may even put us at huge personal risk.

It is worth examining some of the origins of our present societal confusion. The social revolution of the 1960s was an engineered revolution, some of its main protagonists clearly connected to the military industrial complex. 'Sex, drugs and rock 'n' roll' was intended to weaken and scatter young people's wills, harm their bodies and minds, drain their resources, and divide families; ultimately hijacking and neutralising any true grass-roots opposition to the direction of politics. Diets were under-going some massive changes, towards factory-farmed processed foods, filled with toxic chemicals and depleted of vital nutrients. A potent carcinogen and neurotoxin known as fluoride was being added to the water. Mercury and aluminium were added to the vaccines. Polio outbreaks became the scapegoat for a number of things, including neurological harm from the pesticide DDT [2].

An explosion of artistic novelty came out of that revolution as well. But the entertainment industry and media were becoming heavily controlled by large corporations, and any leg-up for the artist now comes with multiple strings attached. In other words, natural human creativity has been co-opted and controlled, just like any other resource.

Medicine had travelled far down the chemical route by the 1960s, and it's fair to say that the scheme to move us away from natural healing systems was already well advanced. The discovery of antibiotics had already sealed medicine's claim to be the only rational healing modality for an enlightened, scientific world. But as far as curatives go, they were one of the very few real tricks big pharma had. And so medical research and scientific publication became ways to make sure people kept seeing chemical allopathy as the natural leader. An entire information industry grew out of that. Propaganda had established itself as a fine art, and considerable scientific effort went into developing sophisticated mind control systems, with countless spin-offs beyond politics and into marketing and advertising [3].

From the 1960s onwards, people were being told *what* to think. By the 1990s, they were being told *how* to think. 'Research methods' became standard in most academic courses. It was no longer enough to have an original idea and follow it through. Now, to get a degree, you have to show that you have followed a defined process from beginning to end, with everything traced back to source. And to get recognition for your findings, you have to get it all peer-reviewed by others who have been through the same brainwashing, and have it published in a journal funded largely by industry. And now Artificial Intelligence (AI) threatens to do our thinking for us, so that there is no way to put a foot wrong with any of the steps.

If you somehow manage to develop something truly challenging to the scientific establishment, then the chances of the public getting wind of it are low, even if they can afford access to the relevant journals. Just as likely, industry will make you an offer you can't refuse and hide your innovations from the world.

The search engine was the obvious tool for making sure people only ever found what they were meant to find. Corporations and governments have whole departments dedicated to managing free resources, both physical and online. Social media turned thinking into a popularity contest, with carefully shaped rules, endemic censorship, and whole armies of professional users, now automated bots. Their job is to manufacture and maintain a zeitgeist within a platform on the one hand, and foment division on the other.

The removal of religion—for all its rights and wrongs—and the alarming decline in first-world fertility, make it much easier to see nothing in life worth taking a real risk for.

Incredibly, we have reached the point where citizens are punished for expressing the wrong opinions. Experts are sent for re-education.

This is where we are—confused, divided, infantilised, and often lacking a clear view on things that really matter. Within this social environment, it would have been very easy to lead us in completely the wrong direction on many things, including our mental and physical health.

Where is the mind?

Does it reside in the brain? I think to a large extent it does, although the mind is far more than the brain, and it seems to extend far beyond the body. Some say it is a transmitter and receiver, linking us with others and to some kind of cosmic database. It may be that and more, but we can't overlook the clear importance of the physical neurology.

The brain is an organ, and a gland, or a collection of organs and glands. And for an organ to function well, it needs support from the body as a whole. A disturbance in its physical environment may therefore disturb its function. In as much as our thinking and processing and homoeostatic regulation can simply go wrong in the brain, it can only be due to bodily disturbance. And so, in both physical and mental disease, we need to look first and foremost to disturbance of the body, and indeed beyond there to the external environment.

On the purely mental side, if the neurology is sound, then disturbance to our understanding of the world can only arise from our environment as well. It is through one kind of unhealthy experience or another that we may become jaded. We certainly can and do hold trauma, with lasting effects that may themselves perhaps be worked on. But the origins of the trauma are 100% external. I don't accept that one can simply think one's way into mental illness and must therefore think one's way out of it.

But the mind does seem to have some kind of homoeostasis of its own. Closure on the past isn't always obtainable, and inevitably we have acquired qualities that can deal with that. An annoying tune does eventually leave the head, unless certain things are happening. Constant reminders will keep it there, and so will *general stress*. Drugs, toxins and certain nutritional deficiencies can also keep us stuck in loops, making change more difficult.

So, we need to look to our experience and any unfinished business for the source of our difficulties, at least as much as to our own thinking. But there is a more general rebuilding that has to take place in order to move on. The actual healing comes through the natural outgrowing of the past. And the things most likely to promote that are a healthy environment and a purpose in life.

In attempting to deal with trauma or ill health through awareness, as we may have to initially, there is a certain need to pull ourselves up by our bootstraps, even if all that means is making the decision to do something new today. And how we may defy gravity thus is surely the biggest mystery, since it can only happen through something called free will. And if the external circumstances persist that led to physical or mental disturbance, then free will has not much else to get its teeth into.

But when disease has noticeably contained some kind of mental element—or even not—the medical and social vogue has, at times, been to look to problematic thinking or localised chemical imbalance as the actual drivers.

Worse, psychosomatics can be the diagnosis of resort whenever the doctor's understanding of the problem is limited. That leaves no room for true causes. The implied answer to mental symptoms, and even somatic ones, can be psychological therapy, or worse, antidepressants. Those solutions are incomplete, at best.

Nevertheless, limiting beliefs can certainly promote and sustain disease. But what I am driving at is that those beliefs can have powerful external and somatic origins. It isn't pretty, but I have to say it: one prime suspect is medicine itself. More particularly, the insistent way that paternalistic medicine owns health and disease, even when it isn't the best fit. It then has to spin its failures as successes in order to sustain its primacy.

There are a number of ways in which medicine can place the blame for failure onto patients, even as it does its very best to help. My belief is, were medicine to loosen its grip even slightly, the burden of first-world disease could be relieved enormously. But with enough awareness, the patient can overcome these social drivers at an individual level. So let's take a look at some of the constructs that are holding us back.

Effects without causes

Modern pain science has somehow led us to a place where there is no physical cause of our symptoms. Through that lens, our pain is probably due to the way our central nervous system is processing information, and not due to pain signalling at all.

By now, you may be able to guess where I stand on this.

The reality is that pain is not some primitive and obsolete sense that can easily be fooled. It is one of our oldest and therefore most highly evolved faculties. It can pick up trouble long before any MRI scanner can. And if we believe pain can mean anything other than that something is wrong, then we are in big trouble.

Part of the problem may be innocent, in that there are technical limitations with imaging neurological activity in vivo. Whatever the reason, the belief that there can be pain without cause is highly dubious. Far more likely is that our understanding of cause is limited.

Another issue is that there need not be actual physical damage or inflammation for there to be pain. And it is true that trouble can be somewhere other than where pain is felt. But that's all a far cry from *absence of cause*, and it's going too far to say that only measurable injury is a valid source of pain. There may well be physical or chemical stress in a so-far unharmed structure, a sort of pre-harm, about which the brain is very aware, and rightly so.

Pain does not have to mean something is broken. It can also mean stop before something breaks. And the more often pain has been felt there in the past, the earlier the warning. This is not a malfunction.

But this all still tries to narrow down pain to source structures, signalling nerves and processing centres, as if that is all there is to pain perception. Even if there is no actual nociceptive (pain) signal detected, the cause is still in the body, and the brain is picking up on it by whatever means and telling us to be careful. The pain is in the brain, only because in one sense it always is. But it's a huge leap to say that it is, therefore, the mind that must be treated.

Where there is true central sensitisation—that is, where the nervous system has become trained through persistent pain, so that pain is perceived long after the cause is thought to have been addressed—there are still other things to account for.

The body is not like the chassis of a car, and the nerves are not simple wires. These are living tissues, and their overall health can be severely compromised by a long-term problem, and by the treatment given. Toxins and irritants can collect from all kinds of metabolic processes. The general idea, that central sensitisation is a specific neurological change, is not adequate, in my view. What is usually missing, when pain persists, is the more general restructuring I mentioned earlier, that needs to take place when stress or bodily insult are over.

Looking at this another way: true chronic pain cases should immediately make us think about some of those other missing links. Show me a case of supposed central sensitisation, and I'll show you a case of prior suppression, that could really benefit from a good healing crisis but has had every symptom quashed.

In support of this idea, I see plenty of acute pain cases, in a context of considerable general stress, where opioids and strong anti-inflammatories have been prescribed. The flaky reasoning is that, in order to prevent them going chronic, the symptoms must be suppressed.

Well, the way to make an acute problem chronic is absolutely to suppress the symptoms. We see it time and time again. It's just that sometimes the patient gets away with it.

Don't forget that inflammation is our most important repair process, and pain is our early warning system. And thus, not only do suppressive approaches prevent resolution, they turn off in-built protective mechanisms (pain),

poison the tissues, and create a dependency on the palliative relief. And, typically, every attempt has been made to
keep the patient's life largely the same as before.

Yet the chronic pain gurus tell us this is pain that persists after the cause has been resolved. It has not been
resolved. It has been displaced into the tissues. In Hering's Law, it has gone deeper (Missing Link 4).

Moreover, pain is a symptom, not a condition. And
thinking about it as a condition in its own right sets us up
for all kinds of confusion.

And still the source of the problem, and its solution,
remain in the body and its environment. Success lies in
approaching them as matters of general health and recovery, not purely as a matter of specific disease and specific
treatment.

Hence, I have seen supposed cases of central sensitisation relieved massively by some pretty straightforward
measures. The only thing I can conclude is that nobody
else managed to figure out the problem, so they gave the
patient a new label. If Cognitive Behavioural Therapy
(CBT) seems to help—currently one of the treatments
offered for chronic pain—then there is a good chance the
reason is some positive effect on overall stress levels. But
it is not enough.

A look at any number of chronic pain websites throws
up some curious contradictions. The explanation of
'chronic pain' is usually given as central sensitisation. But
a big part of the mechanism of therapy is that it alters
one's outlook and behaviour to seek out healthier choices.
This seems to be a backhanded acknowledgement that
our actions, habits and environment have a role to play

in chronic pain after all. The position rather renders the therapy itself redundant, along with the explanation for the cause. Anyone motivated by pain to attend Cognitive Behavioural Therapy is probably going to be motivated enough to cut to the chase if offered a good reason to do so. In other words, they don't need psychotherapy to make them do something helpful: they just need to know what it is that will help.

Is central sensitisation really a problem of strict neurology in that case? The orthodoxy clearly hints at other straws on the camel's back. So what about those? And why does medicine suddenly allow them in now, of all times, when it defines the problem as lacking external drivers? Reductionism has tied itself in knots with this one.

What leaps out, therefore, is that chronic pain remains a general health problem, into which CBT has found a way to insert itself.

The entire thesis of this book is that all health problems are general health problems, and that dissecting them out into directly affected tissues and systems, and most of all not looking for the health, is what causes them to go unresolved in the first place.

True enough, pain pathways can be trained as anything else can. But what I see here is yet another example of medical reductionism failing to get at the sources of suffering, and so inventing another disease. Various kinds of mental health services have grown up around chronic pain problems, for when drugs or physiotherapy are insufficient. And if my position is correct, we will see demand increase, because the results are only partially satisfactory.

There is at least some recognition that general stress can be a major factor in chronic illness, especially pain syndromes. The linear approach of therapy is to calm the nerves or the thoughts one way or another, but without helping the person really sort out the source of their stress. As Phillip Day puts it: "If you have a financial problem, the answer isn't Prozac, it's money." [4].

A large number of modern pain drugs also double as sedatives and antidepressants. They are habit forming, and list effects that you do not want. This approach is bad news for chronic pain sufferers, because once they get a habit for the drugs, getting them out of pain becomes much more complicated.

The witchdoctor says you will die

I was taught in first aid, that if you come across an unconscious accident victim, it's a bad idea to stand over them and say, "I reckon this one's a goner." The hearing is the first of the senses to return, and what they hear in a semi-aware state could tip the scales.

In her book, *Béchamp or Pasteur: a lost chapter in the history of biology*, Ethel D Hume describes a curious case of two sailors bitten by a sick dog at Le Havre [5]. One of the men got all the symptoms of rabies and died within a few weeks. The other one set off for America and knew nothing about it. When he returned fifteen years later he was told what had happened to his friend, whereupon he too developed rabies and died. Another rabies patient began snarling at the medical staff and tried to bite them, being what a rabid dog would do. A doctor then told him that humans with rabies don't do that, they use their fists instead. After that, he tried to punch everyone.

If somebody tells you that you are doomed, the effect can be devastating. In Australia, there was an old practice called bone-pointing, used as a way to enact a death sentence. The person at whom the bone was pointed would quite literally go home and die.

So, what does a cancer diagnosis do to someone taught to fear the dreaded 'Big C'?

We have all heard of the placebo effect. It doesn't mean you feel better because you think you are better. It means you actually get better when you have reason to expect it. And it works both ways: a negative placebo is called a *nocebo*. Likewise, the term 'psychosomatic' doesn't mean the problem is imagined. It means it is a real problem caused by one's mental processes somehow. If the materialists need an explanation, it is that fear raises cortisol levels and thereby affects natural immunity.

But I sincerely doubt there is a disease known to man that somebody somewhere hasn't found a way to recover from. No matter how desperate or difficult the case, there is always something that can be done to make life a little better. We should always offer the patient a reason to recover, and to believe that some improvement, even small, could be possible. Any progress they make, however tiny, should be noticed and valued.

As patients, we should never accept incurability as a diagnosis, and should always be prepared to shop around for answers.

The really curious thing about placebos is that they work even when patients know they are placebos. Most of my own results are due to the placebo effect, so I have sometimes been told. It just happens that my placebos seem to work better than some other peoples' placebos. You can believe it if you want. Homoeopathy also works via placebo, some say. But homoeopathy also works in animals, which is curious, since you can't easily explain it to a horse. A vet once told me it's because the placebo works on the owner. On the other hand, it's possible the remedy works.

Myths of incurability

Incurability can become a self-fulfilling prophecy. I hear things like, "You can't help me—my doctor said it's my ..." followed by the name of the condition. "I've tried everything," is another. Over many years of searching for answers, chronic sufferers can have accumulated a lot of knowledge about what is going on in their bodies, none of which has solved their problem to date. The only hope is an expensive enough doctor or some glamorous intervention.

The difficulty here is not always one of a negative mindset. It can be that there is a strong positive belief in some holy grail of treatment within the disease-based realm. And after many years of searching, resignation to the myth of the condition can be the result. Treatment becomes management and doors start to close.

It puts the therapist in a certain box, too, where medicine lite is readily accepted for peripheral aspects. But some other offer, with perhaps a more general recovery in mind, can be met with incredible resistance. And it's easy to see why. For one thing, there is a sea of offerings out there, many of them wildly simplistic and oversold. Chronic sufferers will have encountered many dead ends, and amateur doctors are everywhere, offering partial knowledge and solutions too good to be true. For another, raising health requires a shift in mindset away from fighting disease. Without taking that step, outcomes are likely to be disappointing.

So it's unsurprising that, when at last a practitioner opens a new door, somebody might choose not to go through. Some patients are ready, and will view the proposal as a breath of fresh air. Others maintain a fundamental faith in the medical way, and it isn't really for us to change that.

So, on the one hand, it isn't wise to oversell. And on the other, nor is it wise to adapt too much to accommodate expectations. Much better to be clear on what we can offer, and the limits within which it might work, and allow our natural audience to find us.

Attachment to the diagnosis

Once a patient becomes resigned to a diagnosis, the very label that once offered hope can become absorbed into their identity. Chronic illness can restructure someone's life, sometimes without them even noticing. And recovery means dismantling their world. I have even heard it said that once cancer is diagnosed, the patient becomes emotionally complete: in some cases it may be true.

Life for the chronic sufferer means more than just surrendering once-cherished activities. It can begin to revolve around clinics and pharmacies and getting blood drawn and all the rest. The allied therapist can become a part of that, and can end up just as dependent on the arrangement as the patient.

Sometimes, for the chronic patient to begin recovery, the first step is to visualise being well. It can be surprisingly hard to see oneself as healthy during a period of sickness. Some are even fearful of trying. But if it can't be imagined, it won't happen.

Financial drivers of chronicity

One of the best predictors of therapy failure is litigation. If there is compensation at stake, recovery can actually harm the sufferer's financial interests. And once obtained, support for a disability can be a much-needed lifeline that healing can threaten. If the patient recovers enough to get their needs assessed at a lower level, they can actually end up in a more difficult situation.

This unintended punishment for recovery is a real conundrum. A civilised society has to support the chronically sick. But any time the sufferer finds himself thinking *I need this money*, he is in really big trouble.

Without equally strong incentives to become well, the support structures for sufferers can become a kind of chronicity machine that keeps them trapped in poor health. I have seen people endure hugely counterproductive programmes because of funding. The politics of this is huge, but not the point of this chapter; it is just something for which we need to be on guard.

For the therapist, it can be hard enough to overcome the purely clinical drivers of chronicity, and the social and financial ones can be impossible. Add into this the financial incentives for the business and we can easily see why so many practitioners thrive on maintaining chronicity. It's not that they intend to keep their patients sick, it's just that the ones who choose to work outside the established frameworks may find it harder to stay in business. In my view, healing will always therefore be a small niche within the so-called healing industry.

Sometimes, the only ethical option is to refuse to join in the dance and hope that the patient may eventually be ready. Meanwhile, any support we offer must at the very least encompass the possibility of some recovery.

When societies lose it

It isn't just individuals who are vulnerable to placebo and nocebo. Whole societies are. We no longer need to wonder what happens when public health systems spread fear and panic, and the media have a lot to answer for. There's a deadly virus going around, nobody is safe, hide inside, and do as you're told. Fear your family, your neighbour, your customers, the people next to you on the train. You've got a cold? That sniffle could kill you. It could kill Grandma! Quick! Line up for testing, even if it means standing in the rain.

It's enough to make a healthy person sick. Long before COVID was a word, there were cases of whole hospital departments getting sealed off because somebody coughed, then everybody felt sick and got tested.

A couple of tests came back positive and faster than you could say, "Don't panic," a deadly emergency was declared, that later on was found to be a figment of everybody's imagination [6]. The phenomenon even has a medical name—*pseudo-epidemic*.

I have met so many people lately who said they know they had COVID, because they were flattened by it, as if they have never had flu before, or had forgotten what the flu can be like. They say it was different, in some way. Yes, it was. What was different was they believed they had something different.

Then there is the other side. The government is lying. There is a power grab under the cover of a global emergency. They are trying to kill us all with vaccines! Whether or not there is any truth in either side, the most important thing is not to let this stuff into the soul. If honest, most of us would admit to losing our minds at some point since 2020.

Reversion to prior learning

Pilots and soldiers sometimes need to replace an old skill with a new one, as techniques improve and standards change. With much training and repetition, they get good at the new way and soon forget the old. That is, until somebody starts shooting at them, and then the old patterns take over and they respond in the old way.

I have met plenty of people who do exactly the same thing when they are sick. Normally they might be sceptical about disease, certain that the answers lie in good health and sensible management of sickness, and insist they would need to have a bullet in their leg before going to hospital. They know something is wrong with medicine and devote their lives to alternatives. Then they get sick while on holiday or something and get nervous about it. Their friends usually spook them the most. Suddenly, they are completely on board with a medical diagnosis and off to the pharmacy with the prescription. It can be like talking to a completely different person. Months of good progress can come undone that way.

A teacher and friend of mine, for whom I give big thanks for helping me see all disease, including cancer, in a completely new light, emailed me after a year or two of silence. He told me he had cancer, and was on his second round of chemotherapy, that it was caused by a virus, and that he was now agonising over whether to get his children immunised. I didn't know what to say. He had the diagnosis, and it was like a switch got flipped. He passed away a few months later. Whether he could have been saved, I wouldn't like to guess.

None of us are immune

I had my own near-brush with the medical system fairly recently due to an inflamed knee. For days it hurt more than a broken bone, but it didn't start out as particularly serious. Had it been managed by combative palliation, I believe it could have become very serious.

It took huge mental presence not to resort to medical help, since I was far from home with few resources. Friends near and far urged me to go to hospital, some using horror stories as persuasion. Even as things started to improve, I nearly panicked and called for an ambulance, suddenly thinking about infective arthritis, antibiotics, systemic complications, and all the rest. A big part of me knew this was all wrong, but the fear nearly took me over.

What kept me going was thoughts of my patients, the ones who had been through even worse and come out the other side just fine. To give in would have meant giving up on everything I believed. Equally important, I didn't like where hospital treatment for crippling inflammation had led others. One friend with a near identical presentation had taken the medical route and ended up with a knee replacement. As it was, I stayed away from hospital, my wife and I nursed it ourselves, the problem resolved completely and, in record time, and my faith was strengthened. True, a sample size of two is not very scientific, but I am glad to have been in the 'control group' that time. But there is nothing like fear and pain to make one rethink everything.

The good news—I repeat—is that these things can work both ways.

[1] David Gillespie, book, *Taming Toxic People*.

[2] Suzanne Humphries and Roman Bystrianyk, book, *Dissolving Illusions*.

[3] Vance Packard, book, *The People Shapers*.

[4] Phillip Day, book, *Little Book of Attitude*, Credence Publications.

[5] Ethel D Hume, book, *Béchamp or Pasteur: a lost chapter in the history of biology*.

[6] Gina Kolata, *Faith in Quick Test Leads to Epidemic That Wasn't*, New York Times, 22 Jan 2007, https://www.nytimes.com/2007/01/22/health/22whoop.html.

A personal position on end-of-life care

It is now more than fifty years since the so-called 'War on Cancer' was officially declared. In that time, we have seen a monumental economic and social effort devoted to defeating this most feared class of diseases. Great promises have been made, and many doctors, scientists and entrepreneurs have feathered their nests lavishly on those promises. Countless billions in public donations and taxes have been poured onto the start-ups and universities devoted to it all.

The effort has been successful, we are told, because we now know more about cancer and have many more ways to treat it. The trouble is, suffering and death from cancer are now far more widespread than before this war began. Many more of us will be diagnosed with cancer and have it written on our eventual death certificates. And the treatments themselves can be horrific.

But people are surviving longer with cancer, apparently, thanks to early diagnosis. Well, in a way that could be true. This sleight of hand would make us think the burden of cancer has been eased, and that we are well on the way to beating it altogether. But the key phrase here is 'after diagnosis'. More people are surviving 'after diagnosis' because more people are being diagnosed, including many for whom their cancer would never have been a problem had it not been discovered. And yes, *from the point of diagnosis,* they may be living longer, but perhaps due simply to the clock starting earlier. This is a far cry from saying medical science is giving people back their lives.

If we make it into middle age as we should, most of us will have one or two things in us that could be called cancer or pre-cancer, that will make little or no difference to our lives or deaths. And unless they become clinically apparent, it might be better not to know. Screening people and diagnosing them without any clinical reason is potentially very dangerous. Yes, if something is wrong, get tested within reason, but otherwise it might be better to think twice.

Furthermore, many cancer treatments in fact follow misdiagnosis, putting people through hell and shortening their lives for nothing. Studies for diagnosis of breast cancer in particular give estimates of anything up to 54% overdiagnosis, but it is notoriously difficult to know for sure [1]. If that is the case, then many of the claims for lives saved are unjustified. And if the same pattern exists for some other cancers, then the benefit to society of their treatment is likewise exaggerated. This also assumes that aggressive cancer treatment actually saves lives, but it's very hard to find an untreated control group to say so.

I have met enough people who have treated their own cancers very successfully to know that it can be a reasonable option, although they have sometimes been shocked at how much the medical system was against them doing so.

The bottom line is, cancer hasn't gone away, it has gotten worse overall, no thanks to advances in medicine.

We can see similar patterns in all the other major dreaded diseases: huge amounts of money poured into solutions and not much tangible output besides symptom management, while the treatments themselves have caused much suffering and medical dependency. Heart disease hasn't gone away, it's getting worse, no thanks to statins. Lung cancer is still a huge problem, despite the war on smoking.

Neurological degeneration, arthritis, inflammatory bowel disease, autoimmunity, asthma—and the list goes on—are still with us more or less as much as ever. Dementia in the old and autism in the young have exploded. More than half of all children in the USA have some kind of chronic condition now. Frankly, medicine is still completely baffled by the common cold, yet still they tell us that the solutions for all these problems are just around the corner ... just keep running the marathons and paying them billions.

But more people than ever are making it to 100, thanks to medical science, it seems. But are they? Almost all the noteworthy advances in life expectancy have been due to other things besides medical treatment. If we remove birth complications and infant mortality from the picture, life expectancy hasn't really changed that much in recent generations. The main advances have been in better nutrition, sanitation and urban design, and in recent decades, preventing accidents. If this is the pattern, then most likely more people survive into very old age simply by living in care homes, where they aren't allowed to fall off ladders while changing lightbulbs, and not because of statins and yearly flu shots.

After all this time, all this effort, all that money spent, what truly, unequivocally effective solution has triumphant medical science finally brought us? Physician Assisted Dying—euthanasia thrown into soft-focus by various euphemisms. You won't get a clearer signal of failure than this. Where has all that effort and public money gone, and what has it really achieved? Instead of clamouring for access to medical suicide, shouldn't we be demanding an audit? I think so.

In the UK, at least, the minds of the population have been seeded with ideas such as it is cruel to let people suffer, and questionable terms like 'dying with dignity'; as if dignity means asking the same people who didn't save you to kill you, without so much as letting your naturopath into the building. The population in Britain is very mixed on the subject, and euthanasia won't be openly legalised any time soon I would bet. It won't need to be. It is already happening, and barely by stealth; it has been legitimised by so-called pathways to relieve suffering towards the end.

If anybody is so deluded as to think this does not amount to the wholesale killing of people before their time, then they aren't awake. I have personally witnessed the extraordinary pro-activeness of the medical system in getting people onto these pathways. I will spare the reader specific examples, but once seen, it cannot be unseen. The chances are that most already have some personal familiarity.

Occasionally, we catch a glimpse of how widespread it really is. Officially, Britain's biggest serial killer was a doctor called Harold Shipman, a GP who died in prison after killing hundreds of elderly people with morphine. The press and the medical system placed the blame on one insane loose cannon with a god complex, drunk on the power over life and death.

But Shipman was small-time. In 2018, the Gosport Enquiry revealed that an entire hospital network in the south of England had been involved in wholesale involuntary euthanasia, and the victims were so numerous that the total might never be known. A handful of staff were implicated directly. Other associated healthcare staff have stated they were involved unwittingly or through circumstance. But whatever their reasons, they had a duty towards the vulnerable in their care. And if they could let it happen, then many more staff of Britain's biggest employer could do likewise.

If somebody really does want to die, or to be numbed against their pain knowing that it might hasten their demise, and they possess complete self-determination, and have at every stage been offered every other possible option, then I won't argue against their values. But how often is that the case? But the really big elephant in the room is that the NHS has systems for it. They have specialists in it. They have service providers who make a living out of the products and training. They have budgets for it. That some quite ghoulish characters are drawn to working in that field shouldn't surprise us.

In Canada it is far worse, so it seems. The problem has got so bad that one Canadian charity has launched a Do Not Euthanise (DNE) registry, and now offers 'guardian angels' for the sick, to watch over their care [2]. Euthanasia is 'available' for not just the terminally ill, but the disabled, minors with one problem or another, and mind-blowingly, the very poor. One comment I heard was that just about the only people in Canada not eligible for euthanasia are the suicidal. The limits of what that society could stomach were only reached when doctors refused to provide it for the mentally ill, as if we are to believe this means there is a conscience in the system after all. It gives some idea of how far off the rails the most caring of professions can go when a society loses its collective mind.

This has been a proud industry in parts of Europe for so long now that one barely bats an eyelid. But the only real difference I see is the degree to which it has been openly legitimised.

I could go into the many possible reasons why this is happening. The monopolisation of medicine for the last century is what has actually led us to this point, but there is a much bigger political picture that I won't labour.

Far more important right now is that people start to realise there is something very wrong with the picture. The justifications don't add up. We are placed on this pathway before birth, not near the end of our lives, and it is up to each and every one of us to decide to get off it. Our very earliest engagements with medicine set us up as customers for medical care by a very limited range of providers, and this is where their provisions can eventually lead.

Many real cures have been suppressed, and the ways to truly stay well have been hidden from us. The drug industry is a branch of the chemical industry that delivers the same products that make us sick. Early detection is the best prevention, we are told, which is nonsense, since something that is detected hasn't been prevented. It is more accurate to say that early detection is sales. Medical detection of early heart disease leads only to medical options—statins, diuretics, blood pressure medication, anticoagulants—none of which definitely improve our life expectancy, and all come with drawbacks.

If we get cancer, we are offered surgery, chemotherapy, or radiotherapy, and little else. Doctors worldwide who dare venture into other approaches risk getting struck off or even put in prison and usually have to work overseas. In other diseases, they can work in the open, but the playing field is tilted against them. In many countries, alternative doctors dare not get too well known, since they risk getting destroyed professionally. I once met a French chiropractor whose own father had been put in prison twice for practising chiropractic.

Cancer patients who want better have to travel to Mexico or Thailand, if they can get there, and they get no help from the state or their insurance companies. Once the elderly get into a care home, the state can take their assets, so that their chances of ever leaving again are tiny, even if they somehow regain their independence under that system.

Even the hardiest of individualists can face so much pressure to take medication for their health, that they may agree just to keep the peace. When the system eventually gets its hands on us, as it will for most at some point, choice becomes very limited indeed. I was recently denied access to a patient on my books who was in a care home, even though she had requested my presence, and

I was offering nothing extraordinary. The reasons given made no sense.

I have known people be given absolutely bewildering treatment in hospital, without any semblance of informed consent, and denied viable alternatives. I have known doctors completely fail to consider the possibility that new symptoms might be iatrogenic—that is, caused by their care. I have known them flat out refuse to help patients find a way off their medications, even when doing so might open the door to other treatment approaches. I have known patients to be warned, for no good reason, against seeking alternatives.

And I have seen how institutions have their own immune systems, capable of exhausting and dividing family members striving to turn the ship around. I have seen every element of this arrangement held up as procedural rectitude and clinical excellence. Those who haven't witnessed all this, and even some who have, will praise and defend the system.

On the one hand, it appears we have more choice in how we end our lives, as if we never had plenty of options for that before. *What the system does not allow us is choice in how we save ourselves.*

Even if we find some other way to deal with disease for ourselves, we can expect very little help and a great deal of opposition.

As far as I am concerned, it is absurd pushing for choice in death until we have dealt with the issue of choice in staying alive.

[1] Tanne J H. *Breast cancer is overdiagnosed in one in six or seven cases*, finds large US study BMJ 2022; 376 :o581 doi:10.1136/bmj.o581.

[2] Frank Bergman, *Canadians Begin Hiring 'Guardian Angels' to Protect Hospital Patients from Euthanasia*, Slay News, https://slaynews.com/news/canadians-begin-hiring-guardian-angels-protect-hospital-patients-euthanasia/.

Postscript

There are no rules, only principles.

—John Wernham

Put another way, in complex systems, rules exist only on a micro-scale, and quickly break down when applied to systems as a whole. That means there is no set of levers that can ever produce wholly consistent results in living patients. Far more realistic and hopeful is to aim for a state of greater stability, and trust that the intelligence of the body will always act towards its own survival, even if it sometimes scares the heck out of us. The more precisely and directly we try to intervene, the less room there is for that intelligence to act.

As healers, we have a choice.

We can continue in our attempts to control the micro or the macro directly, knowing that whatever our intention, the outcome will sometimes be very far from what is desired.

Or we can embrace the uncertainty of non-linearity and exert as little direct control as possible.

The former approach depends on the hope that soon we will know enough that stability won't even matter, since we will have achieved total control. This is the way of the technocrat, and it also means total control of society. Even if that were ever somehow achieved, the question remains as to what sort of arrangement we will be left with, and how bearable life will be under such conditions. Until medicine achieves that mechanistic utopia, many deadly mistakes and much suffering are inevitable.

In contrast, the latter approach gains considerable power from the emergent intelligence within complex living systems, whether conscious or unconscious, that seeks health despite our efforts and not because of them.

For society to persist and advance, I see no alternative but a complete change of general direction towards health creation rather than absolute control of the sick body. This would require pretty much the dismantling of an entire medical system, and the replacement of hospitals and clinics with places that favour life and health rather than make war on disease using poisons as the weapon of choice. They need to combine the power of emergency care with an absolute focus on the restoration of health, involving everything from the architecture, to the catering, to the lighting, to the cleaning, to the routines, to the sorts of staff who call the shots. If we could get this right, we would see hospitals begin to get smaller, as whole departments achieve redundancy. In the meantime, we have to do our utmost to avoid the places.

The most recent experiment in pharmaceuticals, lasting now more than a century, has failed. It is an experiment in which all of mankind has been enrolled without any remote semblance of informed consent and without any attempt at an overall control group. It has solved problems, of course: but many of which we maybe didn't need to have, and many that it seems to have created. It has done so at a significant cost to individual well-being. In many areas it appears to have failed, but it persists as long as society keeps writing the cheques.

Alas, I don't expect the medical system to see the light and turn itself around, even if, somehow, there were to arise a groundswell of demand for reform. The system has become too big to fail. We have all got swept up in its theories and practices, whether we agree with them or not. That leaves it to us as individuals to reclaim our own destiny, to seek out solutions that accord with our own worldviews, and not be too quick to give our doctors the final word.

As practitioners, we should retain our autonomy of critical thought at all times, even if that risks our livelihoods, since what is at stake for all of us is so much bigger. There are much better ways to do what's right for society than just going along with institutional mores and group-think. As patients, we should assert our freedom to choose, and whenever we feel confined to a certain direction of therapy, remember that there is nearly always another option.

I did not set out to write a book on osteopathic theory. But as the text goes on, it certainly does seem to have moved in that direction. The title came to me when preparing a lecture last year, and then I noticed Henry Lindlahr *(Philosophy of Natural Therapeutics)* had discussed missing links, and so it stuck. Nor did I set out to write a book of polemics. But I don't think we can separate where healthcare is going from the various social forces that direct it.

What I have tried to do is lead the reader through the stages of my own conversion, which just happened to lead towards a particular set of solutions.

Through this journey, I picked up an osteopathic degree, but it could just as easily have been something else. From my particular vantage point, what traditional osteopathy proposed in the 1870s seemed to be of such worth that healers and patients of all persuasions should at least be willing to take a look—if not to learn about bodywork, then for some of its broader message about healing. Not least, that healing is a practical matter that needs to be accessible and that depends on natural laws. And that if it depends on poisons (natural or pharmaceutical), occult knowledge, metaphysics and the supernatural, intense exercise or extreme diets to work, then something is often missing. These guiding principles should apply to any healing discipline, I believe.

Osteopathy grew out of pre-existing thought, so it clearly isn't the only possible way to approach healing. It is simply the context I have found to explain things. Most of these ideas crop up in other fields as well.

All of that said, a handle of some kind on the gross structure of the body is essential, and I say that having seen the resolution of complex physiological problems through structural adjustment, including cases where other worthy systems had failed. Almost anything one does to raise health can benefit patients, but I have seen few who didn't gain something from a physical tune-up (adjustment).

It may be possible to compensate for structural drivers in some other way, but then the hard-to-see traps of dependency and vitality drain can potentially loom. Whether or not an individual practitioner wishes to fill in those gaps is up to them. But when healing systems fail in the absence of structural awareness, I do sometimes see patients searching the outer reaches in vain.

Where this work leads next, I do not know. I am prepared for failure or success, or something in between. I have missed out a great deal, and once one starts listing the obvious missing links, many others beg for a mention. I put away pages of thoughts on things like time, stress versus strain, contraction versus contracture, and much more. I thought about including the Autonomic Nervous System (ANS), but it would have opened the door to a far bigger work on precise physiology. The more I think about it, the more I think that isn't needed, at this stage.

The ligaments perhaps deserved a mention. One could see the skeleton as a web of connective tissue with stiffer elements within it, called bones. The more conventional view, that the skeleton is a collection of bones strung together with soft tissue, has many practical limitations. In manual therapy, it can be more useful to think about drawing out the ligaments than lining up bones and loosening tight muscles. There was a risk of going into great anatomical detail, or worse, discussing precise manual technique, which also wasn't the purpose of this book.

The immune system was mentioned several times, but only in passing. For the same reason as just stated, I decided against making it a link, even though it is widely misunderstood. Once we understand that health is the best immunity, and allow ourselves to trust the body, then we don't usually need to know the ins and outs of the immune system. If we don't trust the body, then no amount of knowledge about the immune system is ever enough.

As holists, we are not trying to 'support the immune system', or any other system. We support the body, and immunity takes care of itself. If one looks at the other missing links in that light, natural immunity has been covered amply for the time-being. Where there has been direct tampering with immunity at a chemical level, specialised help is sometimes needed.

The way I see it, the immune system is not a single system, but it is in everything. And simply put, it is the side of homoeostasis that keeps us clean and orderly inside. To support it, we engage in hygienic living in the old-fashioned sense, that is, obeying nature's laws. This worked for centuries before 'antibody' was even a word.

And if we have a fever and a runny nose, we don't see the immune system as needing help. We see it firing on all cylinders. When we occasionally have to spend a day sitting on the lavatory, we don't call it 'gastro' and then fight the gastro. We see it as our needing to eliminate something, thank the body for having such incredible healing powers, and support it through the process.

And in case it needed repeating, yes, severe diarrhoea can very occasionally require urgent hospital care, mainly to avoid dehydration. Anything more than that, when we get back home, we need to ask ourselves how it was that we got into such trouble. The term, 'ingested germs', doesn't really get to the point.

In short, the immune system was dealt with as it should be—indirectly.

Ethics and practitionership—the art of navigating clinical problems—could also have been chapters, but since they were sort of woven in, the points were made.

Courage is another one. Managers do things right, but leaders do the right thing (source: unknown).

In reality, most people lead fairly conservative lives. We like picking from menu options, but real decision making is when there is no menu to refer to. We look to the authorities or to professional services for every problem we face. In turn, professionals refer to guidelines and standards at the times when we most need them to rock boats. And thus, our natural courage is watered down.

We then indulge in manufactured excitements and prepackaged adventures, while avoiding some monumental challenges that are right under our noses every day. We can easily kid ourselves that those challenges do not exist by wearing blinkers and sticking to a prescribed path. We tell ourselves our hands are tied. I believe this, and not sheer malice, is the usual route to ethical failure in institutional staff. In broader society, it is the crucial enabling factor in tyranny.

Then there is the courage in the patient as well, but in a way, that was covered.

If I have done my job well then, the reader will begin to see other missing links for himself and will also start seeing how to apply these ideas with his own pre-existing toolkit. He will figure out which other tools are worth acquiring and which are not. There may be those who have already seen what I see but, like me, just needed somebody to show them they weren't dreaming.

I do also want to mention something called Evidence-Based Medicine (EBM), the idea that all clinical decisions should be based on the best available evidence according to an academic hierarchy of truth. It is one of those concepts that has become too big to fail, but perhaps should fail. Strict EBM has, to some extent, already been discredited, not least because the most outstanding physicians weren't willing to deny what was apparent to them at the behest of statistics. It also meant that when things went wrong, the physician could no longer get the blame, and the people who set his guidelines wouldn't have liked that. But still it hangs on, by softening itself into 'Evidence-Informed Medicine', really confirming that an ounce of good sense is worth a ton of data.

These catchphrases have far more influence as selling points for control hierarchies than as true reasoning tools. If anything, they are academics' attempts at gaining unwarranted primacy, when in fact research is at its most useful when it takes a supporting role. If researchers want to lead front line healthcare, they should go into clinical practice. One academic researcher at my college told me, the thing is that if we keep collecting evidence, eventually a picture will begin to emerge. I say we have had a picture for 150 years and he is wilfully ignoring it. And since a good doctor knows to draw upon studies and data when he needs to, the entire concept is as redundant as it is potentially misleading.

Various works have been written about the flaws of EBM, and of its enabling capacity for, essentially, tyranny. It forms part of that direct line I mentioned, from government policy straight into our care, with ramifications that I personally find frightening. Worse still, EBM lets various private corporations share the line. Doctors can become afraid of having an opinion of their own and can project their fear quite persuasively onto patients. It is unclear then who is really treating the patient.

Guidelines were always meant for the doctor, not the patient. Yet doctors can and do sometimes act as if compliance with best practice is the patient's duty towards them. I have letters to prove it. Thus, EBM has indeed worked against some pretty fundamental ethical principles; those of the patient being free to choose, to be offered alternatives, not to be harmed, to be recognised as an individual, and of the doctor working for the interests of the patient instead of to avoid punishment and litigation.

There are, in fact, many possible systems for making clinical decisions, and being evidence-based is only one of them. For instance, practitioner-centred, where the doctor uses his best clinical judgement based on years of training and experience. Or the patient could choose from a menu of treatments. One could even consult an astrologer or roll a die if one wanted, although they wouldn't be top of my list.

My own favourite is a principles-based approach, the subject of this book. One assumes that the body knows what it is doing and is trying to save itself. One considers all observations in that light and then joins in the effort using one's own particular resources.

One could ask a nurse, who often does more to get people better than the doctor. Or one could find out from the patient's favourite natural therapist what help would get them out of the system in the best shape to take matters forward along other lines. Not much chance of that ever happening, mind you. Or one could just put everybody on exactly the same treatment and hope they survive.

The fact is, *there is no evidence* for evidence-based medicine. Yes, you read that correctly. In order to know which is the best system, they would all need to be tested against each other in some kind of randomised trial. Do the patients of the 60-year-old GP fare best? Or the ones who receive the treatment decided by a computer algorithm? Or the ones treated according to the cycles of the moon? The fact is, we don't know. And thus, in my view, evidence-based medicine falls at its own first hurdle, namely supporting evidence. For all we know, it may on average be no better than consulting fish entrails or tea leaves.

Moreover, if Artificial Intelligence has shown us anything valuable so far, it is that algorithmic approaches to complex decisions are anything but scientifically neutral and objective. They are unavoidably tainted by social theories, and risk becoming powerful tools of social engineering, something that medicine never should have become, but clearly has.

There may have been a softening of attitudes about rigid statistical guidelines. Indeed, we may yet see the failure of the hardcore atheist cultists, to convince society that human judgement is a disaster, and that only infallible science can save us. I hope so. Nevertheless, we will likely see an increasing tension between physicians wishing to practise their craft to the best of their ability, and the greater use of cold algorithms in healthcare.

And so, on a final note, it may well be that the patient and the practitioner will become the greatest missing links of all unless we strive to prevent it from happening.

End

Acknowledgements

With heartfelt thanks to the following for their support, inspiration, advice, encouragement and tolerance, leading up to and during this project:

Ruth Graham, Gerald Slarke, Walter McKone, Nicholas Handoll, Robert Cartwright, H., Joshua Lamaro, Phillip Day, Dr Robert Young, Cara Shaw, Sebastian Eck, Brigitte von Bulow, Frank Perez, Sofie Frenda-Briggs, Joel Hampson, Sunday Lucia, Jodie and Michael Wright, Mel Roser, Nid, Becky, John, Louise and Sacha.

www.ingramcontent.com/pod-product-compliance
Lightning Source LLC
Chambersburg PA
CBHW011725020426
42333CB00024B/2732